Split Ends

Short
Stories

by

Jude Roche

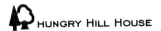 HUNGRY HILL HOUSE

SPLIT ENDS
Short Stories
Jude Roche
Copyright © 1999

Jude Roche
POB 717
Warwick NY 10990

~

The First Nine Months appeared in *Secrets*, 1981

Also by the author:
Words & Selected Verse & Vignettes

~

Editorial Consultant
Margaret A Roche

~

ISBN: 0-7392-0260-X

Library of Congress Catalog Card Number: 99-93287

Printed in the USA by

MORRIS PUBLISHING

3212 East Highway 30 • Kearney, NE 68847 • 1-800-650-7888

~ *Dedication* ~

*To all
who read
these pages*

&
Lovey

≥●

Sweet are the uses of adversity.
William Shakespeare
As You Like It

~ *Contents* ~

~ *Introduction* ~

. . . I saw my mother sitting on the one good chair
a light falling on her from I couldn't tell where . . .

Edna St Vincent Millay

These stories will lead you into the shadowy pathways of
forgotten souls who no one seems to notice and whose troubles,
like silent ghosts, go unseen and unattended to . . . but for the
grace of the author with *a light falling on her.*   **Suzzy Roche**

❧

My mother has been writing stories since she was a little girl,
tending the flame of her creative talent throughout a lifetime of
resistance. By her example, she taught me that the place which
art comes from has nothing to do with fame and fortune. This
premise has enriched my own life immeasurably. The publication
of these stories is long overdue.   **Terre Roche**

❧ ❧ ❧

My sincere gratitude to all who've graciously contributed to the
publication of this book; especially to Maggie for her enthusiastic
support and for proofing tirelessly into the wee hours.

Jude Roche

~ Etude ~

The Depression was what you blamed everything on. It was the reason Uncle Andy lost his car and it was why my best friend, Peggy, had to move away. It was *The Depression* that ended my piano lessons and caused Mr Riggs-Carlysle to fall out of his office window downtown. And it was the reason our father didn't go to work anymore.

It was strange having our father home all the time. We were used to seeing him at breakfast in his good suit with a white shirt and striped tie and smelling of shaving cream, and he'd always have something funny to say before he kissed us all and went out to catch the downtown trolley. Now, he came to breakfast in his Saturday clothes, except for once in a while when he dressed up to go some place called The Interview.

At first, it was fun having him home because he did a lot of fixing and he let us help with the big jobs, like hammering nails and fishing wires down through the attic; or he'd send us to the store and let us keep the penny change.

He found a couple of orange crates and some two-by-fours and showed us how to make skate boxes and then all the kids in the neighborhood made skate boxes and we had a fine time racing up and down the block. Skip McMahon found a can of green paint in his cellar and painted a big Number 1 on the front of his skate box. He and my brother Petey had a fist fight over that because Petey thought his should be Number 1 since he had his first. But Skip had already painted his and Petey took Number 3 rather than follow Skip with Number 2.

Our mother, on the other hand, seemed annoyed that our father was home. They argued whenever they talked to each other and she developed the habit of humming to herself when we were all together so she wouldn't have to talk to any of us. She didn't smile much any more and the least little things got her mad, like a rip in a pair of pants or the hem hanging out of my dress; or the time Petey found a cat and let it sleep in the cellar. "How did I know he was gonna have kittens?" Petey pleaded, but our mother was so mad she cried.

Petey and I examined the new conditions at our house.

"It's The Depression," Petey analyzed. He was ten, a year older than I.

"I don't think I like The Depression," I said.

"Why not? It's fun having Dad home."

"Yes, but it makes Mama cranky."

"Yeah . . ."

"And Frankie Miller says the electric company shut off their lights because they couldn't pay their bill."

"Yeah, but Frankie says it's more fun doing homework by candlelight. He says the candles make spooky shadows on the walls and it feels like a haunted house."

"What's so fun about that?" I asked.

"Well, *you'd* be scared, but I wish they'd shut off our electric."

Then, there was the shopping at the chain store. Every Thursday, we'd go with a grocery list to the chain store a couple of blocks away in another neighborhood. We'd wait while the clerk read over the list and stacked cans and boxes into cardboard cartons to be pulled home by us in Petey's wagon. He'd pull and I'd push up the hill and if we were lucky, only some of the cans would spill out from our load. Once we lost a carton of eggs and Petey went back to the store for another, but the clerk chased him. We had to report the loss to our mother and that was unpleasant because it made her cry.

"Why do we have to get our groceries from the chain store anyway?" I asked Petey.

"Because," he said, "everything's *free* at the chain store."

"But it didn't cost any money at Mr Brogan's store either and it's only around the corner," I said.

"No," Petey explained, "at Mr Brogan's you could *charge* things; that's not the same as *free*."

"Mr Brogan never charged us anything except for candy," I said.

"You just don't understand," Petey explained. "We're *on relief!*"

"What's relief?"

"How should I know? It has something to do with The Depression."

The highlight of our week was our Friday trip to the bread factory. After school, Petey and I would go with a large shopping bag to the big commercial bakery where we could buy day-old bread for four cents a loaf. Even though it meant lugging our books twice as far and waiting in line when we got there, we looked forward to it. Just standing there smelling the fresh-baked bread made us starving hungry and we usually nibbled up half a loaf on the way home.

The adventuresome part was crossing through the railroad yard. Down behind the school and across one of the main roads that led out of town, through an open field that was sometimes swampy, we'd come into the railroad yard with its rows of tracks going east to west as far as we could see. There were always boxcars standing on the tracks and Petey and I would wonder about them, never daring to go too close because we had been warned not to dawdle in the freight yard.

"Bums live in there," Petey told me.

"What are bums?"

"Bums are men who don't have jobs and who live in boxcars," Petey explained.

"Daddy doesn't have a job. Is he a bum?"

"Stupid! Does Daddy live in a box car?"

"But why would anyone want to live in a boxcar instead of a house?"

"Because they like it. Bums can live anywhere they want to. I'm thinking of being a bum when I grow up."

Once, on the way to the bakery, we saw a man hop out of a boxcar and relieve himself. I let out a gasp and Petey clapped his hand over my mouth. We stood very still, afraid that if he saw us, he'd kill us. He didn't though. He climbed back into the boxcar and we ran.

"That's one of the good things about being a man," Petey boasted. "You can stand up to take a leak. I guess that's why there aren't any lady bums. Girls have to have bathrooms and everything just so."

"Well, who wants to be a bum anyway?" I retorted, although, in those days, I wanted to be whatever Petey wanted to be.

When it turned cold and the furnace was operating, we closed off the rest of the house and lived in the kitchen to save coal. It was a big square room with a round table in the center and cupboards all around. Our mother cooked on a big black stove in which she kept a fire going all the time. There was always something cooking, usually things Petey and I didn't like much, but we soon learned not to complain lest our mother cry or our father scold, and we struggled through the casserole to get to the dessert. There was always plenty of bread and butter, and jelly in giant, unlabeled cans from the chain store.

We slept in the bedrooms upstairs and it was so cold, it was just like sleeping outdoors; but we'd dress and undress in the kitchen and run up the stairs and dive into bed, burying ourselves under piles of blankets, with only the tops of our heads sticking out. In the morning, we'd duck out of bed and hurry to the kitchen where our mother already had the stove fire going and our clothes warming beside it, and hot oatmeal cooking. And a nice thing about that stove was that we were allowed to toast the bread over the open fire and it would have a black, burnt taste we didn't like, but we ate it anyway because it was fun to toast the bread that way.

Just before Christmas, we had our first big snowstorm. Our father shoveled the sidewalk in front of our house and heaped the snow in great piles that were over our heads. We'd climb them and slide down until we had shiny grooves worn in them and all the kids in the neighborhood stood in line to take a turn. Our mother complained about so much noise and about not feeling well and our father put his arm around her shoulder, patting her.

"Let them play in the snow, Edie," he said. "It's one of the few things we don't have to buy."

It snowed off and on for two days. It was late in the afternoon of the second day that a man came to the back door with a shovel balanced over his shoulder and asked if he could do the walk for twenty-five cents. Mother shook her head no-thank-you, and the man smiled politely and turned away. But Father couldn't help seeing the man's face all red with the cold, his eyes watering and his nose dripping, and one nearly blue thumb poking out from a worn leather glove. He handed the man a quarter and told him to go ahead. Mother's eyes filled up and she began to hum.

"I know that man," Petey said. "He's a kid in my class's father. How come he's shoveling our snow, Dad?"

"To make some money, son," Father said.

"But Philip says his dad works at the Jansen Store selling men's suits."

"Not many men buying suits these days," Father said, and added, "or anything else."

He was getting more like our mother, not much fun anymore. He would sit, looking out the window or reading the paper or listening to the news on the radio;

or just drumming his fingers on the table or tapping his foot. As though he was waiting, waiting, waiting. In the meantime, Depression or not, Mother was getting chubby.

In the spring, Petey and I resumed our trips to the bakery for day-old bread. After the first few times, though, Petey seemed to have lost his enthusiasm.

"It's boring," he said one day. "I wish we didn't have to go there anymore."

We were in the freight yard on our way home with our books and the bag of bread. We had already broken into the first loaf and I reached in and took out a slice and handed it to him. He shoved it into his mouth, but he wasn't thinking about the bread. He was looking down the tracks at the boxcars.

"Just once," he said, "I'd like to go inside one."

"You wouldn't dare!"

"I certainly would," he said. "You're the sacredy cat."

"I am not!"

"Then, let's!"

"Mama says not to . . ."

"We'll just climb up and peek in," he said. He started down the track, pulling me along.

"What if there's a bum in there?" I asked.

"There's not. I just saw him leave."

"Maybe there's another one, his friend . . ."

"Bums don't have friends. They each have their own boxcar," Petey said with authority. It never occurred to me how Petey knew all the things he knew. I just believed him.

As we approached the boxcar, my heart was pounding. I kept close to Petey who went first. I was surprised to see how big a boxcar was when you got up close to it. This one was orange with big black numbers on its side. When we were quite near it, we set down our books and the bread and walked very cautiously to where the opening was.

"Come on," Petey whispered. "I'll boost you up."

"No, you go first."

Petey climbed up and looked into the car.

"It's empty. Come on." He took my hand and pulled me up.

"It's dark," I said when we were standing at last where we never thought we'd have the nerve to be.

"Well, there's nothing scary about it," Petey observed. "It's just an empty boxcar."

"Hey, look," I said, "there's something in the corner."

We knelt down to look.

"It's a violin case," I said, reaching to pick it up.

"Don't touch it," Petey warned, grabbing my arm. "It could be a machine gun. Gangsters carry them in violin cases, you know."

"Look, there's a book bag, too."

"That's not a book bag, Stupid, it's a brief case. It's probably got stolen money in it."

"Well, shouldn't we rescue it?"

"I'm not sure," Petey said thoughtfully. "What a neat place to hide it, in a boxcar! If it *is* stolen loot and we take it to the police, there might be a reward and we'd get our picture in the paper."

"But we don't know if it is . . ."

"We have to open it," Petey decided. He lifted the brief case and unclasped it. "It's only papers," he said, disappointed. "And somebody's shirt . . ."

"Let me see . . ."

He handed me the brief case and I reached inside it, pulling out the papers carefully so I wouldn't muss the shirt. I leaned toward the light.

"It's music," I said and began to giggle. "That's no machine gun, Petey. It *is* a violin. Open it and see."

Petey, still kneeling, opened the case and, sure enough, it contained a violin. Stamped on the inside of the case were the letters *WPA*.

"I wonder who WPA is . . ."

"I don't know," I said, shuddering, "but if he catches us in here, he'll murder us."

"Shucks," said Petey. "What good is crummy old music?"

"It's kind of funny music," I said. "It looks homemade."

Petey looked over my shoulder, only mildly interested. Music was not one of the things he knew. I, on the other hand, had taken piano lessons. We read the title on the top of the page.

"What's e-tude?" he asked.

"It's pronounced ay-tude," I said, reading *Étude in the Key of H*. "That's funny . . ."

"What's funny?"

"The key of H. There is no key of H."

"What're you talking about? What's the key of H?"

"That's just it," I said. "There's no such thing as the key of H. It only goes up to G."

"So what of it? Is it valuable or something?"

"It's impossible," I said, with authority.

"What is impossible?"

Both Petey and I gasped, for we had not seen the

face looking in at us. In another moment, a man had swung himself up into the boxcar and was standing over us with his hands on his hips, looking very threatening.

"What's impossible?" he demanded.

I couldn't speak, I was so frightened. I moved closer to Petey. The man clapped his hands together as though they were cymbals and shouted,

"Speak up, young lady! What's so impossible?"

"The . . key of H . . ." I stammered.

He began to laugh, hunching down on the floor beside us.

"Do you know music, little lady?" he asked in a gentler voice.

"A little," I said. "I know that there's no key of H."

"Maybe there is," he said. "Maybe there is and we just haven't found it yet. Like the moon. Ever think of that?"

"Sure," Petey agreed.

Abruptly, the man stood up, becoming an adult again.

"Hey, what're you kids doing here anyway?"

Petey gulped. "We weren't going to steal anything," he said. "We just wanted to see what it was like inside a boxcar."

"Have you got anything to eat with you?" he asked.

"Bread," said Petey. "Outside. I'll get it."

Petey leapt up and jumped off the side of the car, leaving me with the stranger. He sat down, settling himself against the wall of the boxcar and smiled at me. He was old, about thirty, and he needed a shave. His suit didn't look bad, a little dusty and wrinkled, but he wasn't wearing a shirt. The shirt in the brief case must have been his only one.

Petey climbed back into the boxcar with a whole loaf of our mother's bread and gave it to the man.

"Thanks, lad," he said, tearing open one end of the loaf.

"I think we'd better be going," Petey said after we watched the man gulp a slice of bread.

"No - wait!" He reached out and held Petey's wrist. "Let me tell you about the key of H."

I realized then that I had been holding the music in my arms all that time. Now, I held it out to him.

"Someday . . ." he said, " . . . tomorrow or the next day or the day after that. It's what isn't yet but what you *hope* will be. That's the key of H. The key of hope."

Petey and I looked at each other, worried. He looked into our faces, expectantly.

"Don't you see? H is what comes after. After G on the scale, but also after *The Depression*. The key of H is having faith, looking beyond . . . to where you're going and what you *can* become. The key of hope, little people. We must all sing in the key of hope!"

He reached over and lifted the violin from its case, settling it gently under his chin. Then, taking the bow, in a long, graceful sweep, he drew it across the strings in one shrill sigh. And as we stood, afraid to move, he played for us his *Étude in the Key of H*. It was the first time I'd ever seen a violin played or heard the sweet, true tones filling up the air around me. And as Petey and I stood frozen in wonder, something about this shirtless man in the dusty suit, cradling his violin, speaking to it from somewhere inside him, made me want to cry. We did not move. He lifted the bow, held it aloft for just a second, then, holding the violin by its neck at his side, he bowed.

Petey and I looked at each other again and then I began to clap and Petey did, too, and the man looked proud and said, "Thank you, thank you." When he had put the violin away and stuffed the music back into the brief case with the shirt, he faced us.

"Go home now," he said. "And no more hanging around in boxcars, you hear?"

On the way home, we talked about it.

"I never thought we'd meet a real bum," Petey said, excited.

"He wasn't a bum. He was a musician."

"Well, what's he doing in a boxcar if he's not a bum?"

"I don't know. Can't you be both?"

"Naw . . . Besides, we were lucky. He could've pulled a knife on us. He talked kind of crazy."

"That's the way *artists* talk," I said. "You're just too dumb to understand."

"And I suppose you do!"

"No, but I know it takes a genius to compose music and play it on a violin. So how could he be crazy?"

"Well, if he's so good, why isn't he in an orchestra?" Petey wanted to know.

"Maybe he will be," I said. "Someday. After The Depression."

We never climbed into a boxcar again and when the summer began, our trips to the bakery stopped.

One day our father shined his shoes and got dressed in his good suit and put on a nice bright tie and went downtown to work. And shortly after that, we got up one morning to find Aunt Jane in the kitchen instead of our mother, and Father told us that Mama was having a rest in the hospital and that when she came home in a week or so, she was bringing a new baby brother with her.

We started buying our groceries at Mr Brogan's store again, and when our mother came home with the new baby, she didn't hum anymore; and she smiled, the way she used to before *The Depression.*

~ *The Grace of a Happy Death* ~

In second grade, I learned to pray for a happy death. Only seven years into life, I pondered death, which had recently befallen both my grandmothers; death, which had occasioned somber visitations to our home by a parade of strangers, and which caused my mother to cry; death, which Sister Joseph Louise seemed somehow to value more than life, thus urging us to pray for its happiness.

A happy death, according to Sister Joseph Louise, was not simply passing peacefully away in one's sleep, but passing away in the state of grace, free of mortal sin.

It was possible, Sister Joseph Louise said, to be a saint, not necessarily a prominent one like Francis or Joan of Arc, but a saint nevertheless, if one died in the state of grace. Everybody's mother was a saint. God, it seemed, held mothers in special esteem. It was comforting to know one's mother was slated for sainthood and that the very condition of motherhood assured her of a happy death. No such assurance was provided for fathers, however, and since my father took a drop now and then *and* the name of the Lord in vain, it was for him and the grace of his happy death that I prayed.

Of course, I wanted to be a saint, too, and I practiced being very good so that God would reward me with motherhood. I did not talk in church, nor turn around, for that was like slapping God in the face. I tried to avoid having impure thoughts, although I wasn't quite sure what they were. I got good grades and was considered an obedient child. In the May procession that year, I was runner-up to Patricia Riley in the competition to crown Our Lady. Although my grades were better, Patricia, with her golden curls, looked more like a Madonna than I, and her father was active in the Holy Name Society.

In sixth grade, I learned about virgin martyrs. They were young women who achieved their sainthood by yielding their lives rather than their virtues. Although the process was never really spelled out, we envisioned a young Sister Joseph Louise resisting the advances of a hulking male, her flesh clawed to shreds, her limbs torn asunder and herself left to perish happily in the state of grace. Why a hulking male should wish to assail an innocent like Sister Joseph Louise was beyond our comprehension but it served to buttress advice our elders gave us about accepting candy or rides from strangers.

Babies, if they died, became angels and lived happily ever after in the sight of God. Even so, when little Colleen Murphy down the street died of pneumonia, there was much weeping and keening and her parents were inconsolable. Had Colleen lived, she doubtless would have become a mother or even a nun, as did her elder sister, and in either case, she would achieve sainthood. Whether it was more advantageous to be an angel or a saint deserved consideration: angels, when referred to, were *he* or *him*. I wondered, then, if Colleen, when she died and went to heaven, traded in her gender.

While the sisters ran the school under the wing of Mother Superior, Monsignor Donlevy, the pastor, was the real power. We believed that he owned the church and school and that, in a sense, he was king and we, the parishioners, were his subjects. He was assisted by two younger priests, Father Walsh and Father Belli, who heard our confessions on Saturday afternoons and visited our classrooms occasionally, often saying something to make us laugh.

But when Monsignor Donlevy made one of his rare appearances, we thundered from our seats and stood frozen in the aisles, reciting in unison with Sister, "Good morning, Mon-seen-yor!" And so we would stand until he bade us be seated. And the while he spoke inaudibly with Sister, we would titter and twitch until he faced us and asked a question from the catechism to see how many hands would go up in response. I would long to be called on, but dreaded it, too. Monsignor Donlevy, with his long black cassock and biretta, appropriately magenta-trimmed, was an awesome hero, the ultimate father figure, authoritative, sexless.

There was a succession of nuns in my life following Sister Joseph Louise, but it is she I remember most because she was the prettiest. Her skin was rose-creamy and bulged less against her coif than did the other nuns'. She had very blue eyes and she didn't wear glasses, and the graceful arch of her brows seemed to have been lightly sketched in charcoal. Only a straight, definite nose cast its shadow of authority upon the softness of her face. I wondered what color, underneath her veil, her hair had been before it was shorn; and beneath her heavy black habit, did her thighs curve perfectly as did the angels' thighs in the stained glass windows of the church?

Had Sister Joseph Louise noticed me in second grade, I should probably have been called to be a nun. Our class left her behind when we graduated to third grade and it wasn't until sixth grade, when we became choir members, that we were reunited with her.

I was not one of her favorites, though I longed to be. I lived for the moment she would notice me, speak to me, but I was sure she barely knew my name. I suspected she didn't like me at all for she put me in the alto section, so I could never sing melody. I thought my plainness was the reason. I was small and insignificant and my hair was short and straight. My clothes never fit properly because they were handed down from a cousin who grew out of them faster than I could grow into them. I practiced diligently to learn the unmelodic alto parts of the hymns so that Sister Joseph Louise would single me out as a good example. But her praise seemed always directed at the sopranos who, after all, had the easiest part to sing.

I lost my fondness for Patricia Riley when, in seventh grade, she developed breasts and attracted the attention of Dennis Mitchell who I had always thought would become a priest. I lost my respect for him, too, because he took up smoking cigarettes and saying *hell* and *damn*. Of course, he was older, an eighth-grader, but up until the time he discovered vice, he had thought only of football. It was one thing to watch him hugging the ball as he ran down the football field, looking heroic, strong and chaste. It was disgusting to see him with a cigarette in his mouth, hanging around, ogling

Patricia Riley.

In eighth grade, I developed breasts of my own and I was allowed to use the curling iron on my hair. My father disapproved, of course. I suppose he thought I would never have breasts, that my hair would always be short and that I would go on forever looking like my brothers. My being a girl imposed a whole new set of frustrations on him. I was forbidden to consort with boys except in properly chaperoned groups. There was no danger; I would not risk the pains of hell for the adventure of a silly kiss.

By a stroke of luck, Sister Joseph Louise became our eighth-grade teacher. Sister Daniel Marie, so old that she had even taught my mother, was called to her happy death during the summer and when we returned to school in the fall, all the nuns had been reassigned to different classes. Sister Joseph Louise was no longer the youngest of them, but I still thought she was the prettiest. And now, she was to teach us, the seniors.

Some of the more sophisticated among us called her Sister Jo, though not to her face. I preferred the lyrical sound of Sister Joseph Louise which, we supposed, were the names of her parents. We believed that a nun gave up all her choices, all her worldly claims, even to her own given name.

Priests, as we knew them, did not give up their names, nor live in seclusion, presided over by a Father Superior. They did not cut off their hair; and underneath their cassocks, they wore trousers the same as other men. They drove cars and went on vacations and occasionally were invited to dine with families in the parish.

The student fortunate enough to have had Father

to dinner became a class celebrity, for Father's endorsement was sterling. Of course, I enjoyed no such preferment. I had never spoken to a priest outside the confessional and even then, my sins were never exciting enough to promote a conversation. I would race through my *Act of Contrition*, often hearing the slide between us slammed shut before I finished. I wondered what the priest would say to me if I confessed a really mortal sin - murder, or worse, *adultery*, whatever that was. I might have been tempted to try it if I hadn't been so scared. Besides, lying in confession was sacrilegious, which was even worse than adultery.

As an eighth-grader, a senior, I was not as timid as I had been in the earlier grades. It no longer worried me that I was short and didn't have curly hair. I was a good student. I got straight A's, and that, after all, was what finally caught Sister Joseph Louise's attention. Not only did she notice me at last, she actually talked to me about my future and urged me to pray for a vocation. Although I could not tell her so, I did not want to enter the convent.

As we neared the final weeks of school and our long-awaited graduation, Sister Joseph Louise announced what our senior project would be. There was to be a special award given at graduation to the student who submitted the best essay on *My Chosen Career*. Everyone had to participate. To help us along, Sister listed some suggestions on the board, in two groups:

Boys: Priest, Doctor, Lawyer, Policeman, Fireman, Engineer, Soldier/Sailor, Professor, Businessman

Girls: Mother, Nun, Teacher, Nurse, Secretary

According to Sister's list, there were more choices open to boys than to girls. Arthur Gates, who was the smartest boy in the class, wanted to be a lawyer. But Bernard Cusick wanted to be a big-league baseball player and Anthony DeSala wanted to go out west and become a cowboy. I noted, too, that Sister's list for the boys did not include *Father* as a career, even though *Mother* was first on the list for girls.

Angela Russo opted to be a nun, like Sister Jo. Nora Moran thought she'd like nursing, for the noblest of reasons - she'd be helping to save lives. Audrey Harp chose teaching and Jane Swan wanted to be a secretary, but most of the girls preferred motherhood. Patricia Riley, however, surprised everybody by announcing that she wanted to be an actress, specifically, a movie star.

None of the choices on the girls' list appealed to me. I had long ago abandoned motherhood as a vocation, even though it narrowed my chances of sainthood. Being the eldest of six, I had my fill of tending children. We were a close family, fond of one another, but there didn't seem to be much in it for my mother. Her life was an endless performance of one service or another, none of it netting any recognition. She rarely complained, but she was always tired and her social life consisted of attending Mass on Sunday mornings and having relatives to Sunday dinner. Rarely was she invited to someone else's dinner; there were just too many of us.

I didn't feel suited to teaching, although I considered it briefly because teachers had the summer off to travel in Europe. Nursing was out. I had no competence with illness and being a secretary appealed to me least of all.

My Aunt Polly was a secretary, a most proper lady, whose whole life seemed to revolve around a Mr Halvorsen. Her view of the world was filtered through Mr Halvorsen's opinions; her activities were tailored to his convenience. At Christmas, he would give her a five-dollar gold piece and a box of candy. Although Aunt Polly kept company with Mr Canaday who owned a small grocery store in the neighborhood, she wouldn't marry him. He said *ain't* and ate peas off his knife and he drank beer, whereas Mr Halvorsen was a connoisseur of fine wines.

So, Sister Joseph Louise's list of career choices posed a problem to me. I did not want to pursue any of them. I knew that she wanted me to enter the convent. I needed only to write a brilliant essay on my desire to become a nun and I was almost certain to win the prize. But I could not. Much as I loved God - and Sister Joseph Louise - I could not lie to them both, even at the expense of the prestigious award.

I had to think of another field I might enter, something that I would truly like to do and that would also impress Sister Joseph Louise. I considered becoming a newspaper reporter. I had seen a movie once about a lady reporter. She was clever and witty, beautiful, of course, and in the end she married the handsome detective. But she agreed to stop being a reporter when they married, although he went on being a detective just the same.

Women, it seemed to me, were destined to be assistants. In the home, the father was the head of the household. Women were teachers but they were seldom principals. Nurses aided doctors and secretaries were - well, office valets. Sister Joseph Louise, a nun, a woman, could not administer the sacraments or celebrate Mass; yet, I knew of no one who loved God more.

I did not want to be an assistant, so I shifted my attention to the boys' column to find my chosen career. Obviously, I couldn't be a business*man* or a fire*man* or a police*man* or a soldier or a sailor. Professor had a nice ring to it, but a professor of what? Besides, to impress Sister Joseph Louise, my career had to be one that helped me to serve God. It narrowed down to three - lawyer, doctor, priest - solidly male callings.

A lawyer could defend people and protect their property. A doctor could save their lives. But what more rewarding career could there be than to guide them to the grace of a happy death! *I would be a priest!*

That there had never been a woman Catholic priest did not phase me. I was sure that my vocation had been inspired by God. It was a career that would embrace all the virtues Sister Joseph Louise would hope for me - purity, piety and a dedication to God and eternal life. Celibacy was no problem. Since I wanted no children, it was easy to discard marriage, for one without the other was either scandalous or tragic. Besides, celibacy appealed to me far more than virgin martyrdom.

I confided the first draft of my essay to my parents. My mother reviewed it with amusement and sympathy but she felt sure that Sister Joseph Louise could not seriously consider it for a prize, and certainly Monsignor Donlevy would be outraged at such a notion. My father, comforted that at least I was not boy-oriented, thought the whole idea was a joke, especially the part about women hearing confessions when everybody knew they were compulsive gossips.

Nevertheless, I wrote my composition as brilliantly as I could and I presented it three days earlier than the deadline. I felt sure that Sister Joseph Louise would love it. Of course, Monsignor Donlevy would be the ultimate judge, but surely Sister's recommendation would carry some weight.

The remaining days till graduation passed slowly. Even exam week seemed to drag. I passed the finals with ease, confident that I would again make the honor roll. The only element of suspense was the essay contest. It meant more to me than the honor roll, more than graduating, even more than the parties that were planned and the gifts I would receive.

The positioning of my career had made me probe into the hazy, wooded areas of my intelligence. It had forced me to examine concepts that had been neatly packaged and tucked into my head to function as automatic controls. I had sorted through those concepts and discarded the ones that didn't fit and I was excited about it. I fantasized that it would excite Sister Joseph Louise, too; that she would stand with me on the stage, smiling proudly as the assembly applauded me for my ingenuity.

I understood her remoteness toward me during those days. She could not afford to even hint at who the winner would be. Obviously, she was avoiding me so the others would not suspect that I had won.

On Graduation Day, I sat with my classmates in the school auditorium, the girls in white caps and gowns, the boys in blue. On the side aisles our parents had gathered with siblings and dutiful relatives. On the stage, Monsignor Donlevy sat with Sister Joseph Louise, Father Belli and Father Walsh. In the center of the stage was the podium and piled upon it, tied in blue ribbons, were our diplomas. Father Walsh conducted the ceremony, introducing first Miss Angela Russo who delivered the salutatory address. I won the spelling award and was presented with a gold medal inscribed with my initials. There were other awards, too, and Master Arthur Gates finished the program with a valedictory speech, but not before the winner of the essay contest was announced . . .

Father Walsh introduced Monsignor Donlevy and everyone applauded. He stepped to the podium, grasping each side of it with his authoritarian hands, just as he did in the pulpit. He looked out upon us through his bifocals, his face ruddy and smiling. It was his pleasure, he said, to confer a very special award upon one among us for the best essay on *My Chosen Career*. My heart pounded so hard, I thought I would faint. He assured us that it had not been easy to decide from among so many excellent submissions. But a choice had been made and it was with pride and great pleasure that he bestowed upon *Miss Mary Ann McHugh* . . .

. . . and that was all I heard - that Mary Ann McHugh, not I, had won the essay contest. Through the film of tears collecting in my eyes, I fancied I saw them - Father Belli, Father Walsh, Monsignor Donlevy and Sister Joseph Louise - laughing derisively at me from the stage, while my parents, my classmates, the whole assembly thunderously applauded the winner. I saw Mary Ann McHugh hasten to the stage to claim the prize and heard her breathlessly thanking everyone from God on down. I sat in a daze, rigid, drained of all the enthusiasm and excitement I'd had. It didn't matter that I was graduating with honors or that I'd won the spelling medal. *I should have won the essay contest!*

There was more applause as Monsignor Donlevy awarded each diploma. Someone nudged me toward the stage. I mounted the few steps and walked waveringly toward the podium. I had to pass in front of Sister Joseph Louise, Father Belli and Father Walsh. The two priests grinned, apparently amused at my distress. But Sister Joseph Louise studied her hands, folded in her lap. She wouldn't even look at me! I knew then that, instead of making her proud of me, I had embarrassed and shamed her.

I stumbled toward Monsignor Donlevy. I heard him say my name. He handed me the diploma wound in its blue ribbon and extended his other hand for me to shake.

"Congratulations, Miss Ryan," I heard him say.

Like a robot, I reached for his hand and we looked into each other's eyes, mine bright with tears, his hard as agates, frozen in a smug, humiliating smile.

"Good luck to you," he said rhetorically.

And then, as I slumped, fainting, to the floor, I heard my own voice ring out like an echo, saying, as gracefully as it could,

" . . . and to you, Monsignor, a happy death!"

~ *The Summer of James* ~

I was eleven that summer. My two girlfriends were away at camp. My sister was only seven, too young to play with, and my brother was a boy. It promised to be a boring summer. And then, I met Eunice.

It all began with James. He was thirteen and in September he would go to the high school which meant I probably wouldn't see him any more. Not that I saw much of him anyway. Oh, I saw him, but he didn't see me. If he thought much about girls, he needn't have thought about me, for there were lots prettier girls in school than I. But I thought a lot about James. To me, he was beautiful. Especially on Sundays when he served Mass and he stood on the altar in a black cassock and white surplice, with his hands folded together, looking solemn and reverent. I mean it, he was beautiful.

It was no fun going swimming alone, but I went to the park every day just to pass by the house where James lived. I knew a place away from the playground, up a hill where no one else went. There were trees and grass and wildflowers and a whole lot of sky overhead. I would lie in the grass and just think about James. I would fantasize how, on my way home, I'd pass by his house and he'd be sitting there on his front steps and when I went by, he'd say *Hi* and I'd say *Hi* and maybe he'd walk me home. And then, somehow, he'd touch me. I thought it would be delicious if James touched me. I'd make promises to myself as though I were my own fairy godmother. I'd say, *If I hurry along to the big tree at the end of the path before that bluejay flies away, I can count up to three with my eyes closed and when I open them, James will be there.* Of course, I was only daydreaming, but, who could tell? one day it might happen.

And then, one Saturday afternoon, it did happen. I had been to church, to confession. I said my penance and walked up the aisle with my hands folded and my eyes down, so I didn't see him until I got outside. And there he was, just leaning on the railing of the church steps. I thought he must be waiting for someone because you almost never see boys by themselves. I often saw James with his big brother, Kenny, who was in high school and who all the girls were crazy about. I pretended not to see him but I was shaking so that I could just about have fallen down the steps. And then, I couldn't believe my ears . . . just exactly the way I'd planned it a hundred times, he was saying *Hi* and I said *Hi* although I could hardly hear my own voice. I kept right on walking and pretty soon I heard him coming after me.

"Wait," he said, "I'll walk with you." And he fell in beside me. He asked me where I lived and I told him Willow Street.

"It's a hot day," he said.

"Awfully."

"Don't you go to camp or something?" he asked.

"No. How about you?"

"Not me," he said. "I've got a job."

"Really?"

"Yeah. At Errico's Hardware Store."

"Do you wait on customers?"

"Sometimes, if it's very busy," he said. "Mostly I unpack boxes and put the stock on the shelves."

"Maybe I'll see you there sometime," I said.

"Sure."

Now we reached the corner where he would have to turn to go to his house and we slowed down a little.

"Shall I walk you home?" he asked. And he did.

When we got to my house, my parents were sitting on the front porch, so I quickly said, "Goodbye. Thanks a lot. See you . . ." And I ran into the house. I didn't want my folks to meet James and I was sure he wouldn't want to meet them. Once inside the house, I watched him walking away, whistling, with his hands in his pockets.

During the next week, I didn't know what to do with myself. There was no point in walking past James's house since I knew he was working at Errico's. I wished my mother would send me to get something for her at the hardware store, but she didn't and I certainly couldn't just go there for nothing. And so I was just sitting there with a long face thinking about what a boring summer it was.

"Why don't you go across the street," my mother suggested. "I think Eunice has arrived."

Eunice was Mrs Miller's younger sister who was coming to visit for the summer. The Millers had moved in across the street a couple of months back and my mother had taken a liking to them, especially Mrs Miller who was kind of sickly. I had been in their house with my mother a few times and there was a beautiful picture of Mrs Miller in a gorgeous white wedding gown with a train on it that covered the whole floor. In that picture she was as pretty as a movie star. That's how I knew she was sickly because she didn't look like that now. She looked gray and drawn and sometimes, even after lunch, she was still in her bathrobe.

I'd heard them talking about Eunice and they'd already decided that when Eunice came, she and I were going to be friends. Parents do that: they think that just because two kids are cousins or the same age or in the same class in school, they are automatically friends. Well, it doesn't work that way and I wasn't about to dash across the street making friends with Eunice until I got a look at her first.

Two days after she arrived, I finally met her. I was sitting on our front steps when she came out of the Millers' house and straight across the street to ours. I could see right away that she was different. She walked right up to me and said,

"Hi, I'm Eunice. I guess you're Linda."

She smiled and sat down beside me. She looked a little like Mrs Miller in that wedding picture. What I mean is, she didn't look to be my age. She could have passed for sixteen. It turned out she was fourteen and so, when she asked me how old I was, I lied a little and told her I was twelve. I was fairly tall for my age and besides, in November, I'd be twelve.

"What do you do around here for excitement?" she asked.

"Do you want to go swimming?" I suggested.

"Is there a beach near here?"

"No," I said, "but there's a pool in the park."

"Oh," she said, disappointed. "Well, I don't swim. I like to tan, though." She looked at me. "You have a nice tan," she said.

I'd never thought about getting tanned on purpose. It was just something that happened to us every summer.

We went to the park and I noticed for the first time that my bathing suit looked kind of faded. In fact, beside Eunice, *I* looked kind of faded. She came out of the bath house wearing a bright red bathing suit that made her white skin seem even whiter and her curly blond hair jiggled on her bare shoulders as she walked along. Another thing: she had hips and a *bust!*

I left her lying on a towel at the deep end, then I held my nose and jumped in where the water was over my head, partly to show off and partly because I wanted to hide. I was a pretty good swimmer, but I hadn't mastered diving. Right then I was glad I couldn't dive because all of a sudden I knew I didn't have the figure for it. I swam around a little and when I went back to where I'd left Eunice, there were a couple of boys chasing each other around her and diving into the water trying to attract her attention. She was lying there pretending she didn't see them. When I sat down beside her, she sat up and began to giggle. She was actually enjoying their foolishness. After a while, she pointed to the top of the hill, my hill.

"What's up there?" she asked.

"Nothing. Just some trees."

"Let's go up," she said. She jumped up, collecting her things. She ran a little distance from me and shouted back, "Let's climb up that big hill," just as though we hadn't already talked about it. I was aware she wasn't talking to me.

We went to the park every day and it was always the same. The boys would try to attract her attention with their diving and their stalking. She seemed to enjoy their attention, but she remained aloof.

"They're just babies," she said. "They have to grow up."

Then we'd get dressed and climb up the hill and just sit and talk. Besides being pretty, Eunice was smart. She lived in New York City and there were over a hundred kids in her class at school. She went to dances and she knew all about boys, and she was going to be a model when she got out of school.

"Have you ever been kissed?" she asked me one day. "By a boy, I mean."

I shook my head no.

"At the mission," I said, "the priest said kissing's a sin."

Eunice frowned.

"How could kissing be a sin? If people didn't kiss, how could they tell whether they were in love or not? Nobody'd ever get married if it weren't for kissing."

"Did you ever kiss anybody?" I asked her.

"Of course," she said. "Don't you even have a boyfriend?"

I said no. I'd never told anybody about James, not even my two girlfriends. Besides, he wasn't what you'd call a boyfriend anyway. Eunice sighed, disappointed in me.

"You're more of a kid than I thought," she said.

I didn't want Eunice to think of me as a kid. I wanted to suddenly grow up and be like her. I couldn't risk her losing interest in me so I decided to tell her about James the next time we went to the park. The next day when I called for Eunice, she couldn't go to the park. Mrs Miller wasn't feeling well and she'd asked Eunice to stay around the house in case she needed her. So Eunice and I sat on the porch and talked. I didn't want to blurt out about James, so I said,

"I'm sorry Mrs Miller isn't feeling well."

"Oh," said Eunice, "she'll be all right when it's all over."

"When what's all over?"

"The baby."

"What baby?"

That's when Eunice really lost patience with me. "Didn't you know she was pregnant?"

"Pregnant?"

"She's going to have a baby. Couldn't you tell?"

I didn't know what she was talking about.

"Good lord," she said, "Don't you know *anything*?"

She didn't expect me to answer.

"Where did you think babies came from?" she asked.

"I guess I never thought about it," I said. "From heaven?"

That made Eunice laugh. She sat there hugging her knees and laughing as though I had said something very funny.

"Tell me," I said, although somewhere in the back of my mind, I didn't really want to know.

"There's a baby right there inside my sister's stomach," Eunice said, whispering, as though it was a secret. I wasn't sure I heard her right but when I recovered, I asked her how it got there.

"From making love," she told me.

Now, I'd seen love-making in the movies, like

when the handsome hero grabs the beautiful girl and presses her shoulders together until her head bobs up and then he swoops down and kisses her with all his might and it's the end of the movie. But I couldn't quite see my own mother and father carrying on like that and they had us three children. I thought possibly Eunice had gotten the wrong information. But she seemed very sure and she did come from New York and she'd been around, as she said.

"Being in love must be wonderful," Eunice said in a kind of dreamy way. I thought about poor Mrs Miller lying in there feeling so sick and I had my doubts. Then Eunice began to pout and she stamped her foot.

"I wish there was something to do around here," she said. "Don't you know any boys?"

Now was the time to tell Eunice about James.

"There is one boy that I like," I said.

Eunice was interested.

"Really? Is he cute? How old is he?"

I told her the little there was to tell about James but I had to admit that I didn't think he was at all interested in me.

"Why not? You know, you wouldn't be bad looking if you curled your hair." She patted the ends of my hair and then she looked as though she was getting an idea. She was.

"Why don't we go to the hardware store and buy something so I can get a look at him," she said.

"What'll we buy?"

"Anything," she said.

I blushed to think of doing such a thing, but Eunice explained that you have to be forward.

"Boys," she said, "are too shy to make the first

advance."

So the next day we went to the hardware store and bought some flashlight batteries, but James was nowhere to be seen. I was disappointed but Eunice was still determined to stir up something to do.

"Does James have a freind?" she wanted to know.

I told her about Kenny, his brother, who was in high school and who all the girls were crazy about. Then, she really got interested. She was so set on meeting James and his brother that I was afraid she'd actually go right up and ring their doorbell. Of course, she wouldn't really do that, but that's how interested she was. Then I remembered about confession.

"We could go to church, to confession on Saturday afternoon," I said. "Maybe they'd be there. They might walk us home."

"Hold it!" she said. "I've never been inside a church, much less to *confess* anything!"

"You don't have to confess. Just sit there and wait for me."

"What are you going to confess?" she asked.

"My sins," I said.

"What sins?"

I blushed. "Just little sins," I said, "you know, *venial* sins."

"Like what?"

I didn't feel like telling Eunice that my venial sins were sassing my parents or telling a lie or saying *damn*, so I said,

"Sins are secrets you only tell to a priest."

Eunice felt secrets were to be told to your best friend, not to a priest hiding in a dark closet.

"Your religion," she said, "is scary."

34

But she agreed to go with me to the church on Saturday.

"Eunice," I ventured, "do you think you could show me how to curl my hair?"

Eunice did a nice job on my hair. She made my bangs into a soft wave and the rest was all fluffed out like a cloud of smoke. I liked it but my mother didn't. She thought it made me look older than I was. And she wondered why all the fuss about hair when you were just going to confession.

Eunice, of course, looked beautiful. She was wearing a white silkish dress with a skirt that swished about her knees as she walked. And she was wearing high heels and lipstick, too.

When we got to the church, there was a cluster of boys standing on the corner. James and his brother, Kenny, were among them. We hurried past them and went up the steps to the church but when we got to the door, Eunice decided that she'd rather wait for me outside. I'd have been too embarrassed to stand out there with all those boys gaping. But, when I came out of the church, the boys were gathered around her and she was telling them that she was visiting from New York City and that she was studying to be a model. We stood around and talked. That is, I stood around and Eunice talked. Then, at what seemed to be a strategic moment, Eunice announced that we'd have to be getting home. James's brother, Kenny, asked Eunice if he could walk her home and she said yes, of course, and that's how it was - Eunice and Kenny walking together just ahead of James and me.

Afterwards, when the boys had left us on our

street corner, Eunice squeezed my hand.

"I made a date for us for Friday night," she said.

"A date?" I cried. "I'm not allowed to have a date!" I hated to admit it but dating was not even a dream in my immediate future.

"Don't worry," Eunice said. "We're just going to the movies. We'll meet the boys there. Nobody will know we're meeting them and it'll be *like* a date."

The thought of sitting next to James in the dark at the movies for a couple of hours made my heart beat noisily.

For the next four days, I felt wonderful and I felt awful. When I thought of James, I could feel funny little bumpings going on inside my heart and all the way up to my throat. I'd think of how beautiful he looked on Sunday mornings on the altar. And then, without wanting to, I'd imagine something terrible, like James in his underwear, with bow-legs or knock-knees; or James at work, dropping a box of nuts and bolts all over the floor; or James getting bawled out by his father for smoking a cigarette.

Once, my mother caught me staring at her and she asked me what was the matter. Of course, I couldn't tell her, but I was wondering if it was really true that I was once inside her stomach and, if so, how did I get there and how did I get out. I was afraid to ask for fear she'd laugh because the more I thought about it, it really was a ridiculous idea. But I couldn't help thinking about it and when I wasn't thinking about James, I was thinking about *that.* The fact was, I was thinking about James and kissing and babies and the more I thought about it, the worse it got. Sometimes I'd almost cry and then another time, I couldn't wait until it was Friday and I was sitting next to James at the movies. Sometimes, alone in my room, I'd feel myself blush all the way down to my toes. And once I felt so peculiar that I thought I was going to be sick. I told Eunice about it and she understood.

"You must be in love," she said.

When Friday came, I ran into some trouble because my parents weren't going to let me go to the movies at night. But Mrs Miller put it to my mother as a favor since she didn't feel well enough to entertain Eunice herself and so I was allowed to go.

We walked to the movie theater. It wasn't far. We bought our tickets and went inside. We were early, before the lights went out, and we could see that James and his brother, Kenny, weren't there yet, so we went into the ladies' room where Eunice combed her hair and put on some more lipstick. She said I could use some if I wanted to, but I didn't.

James and his brother, Kenny, were just arriving when we came out of the ladies' room. My heart started all that bumping again and I felt like running right out of the theater. Eunice looped her arm through Kenny's. He offered to buy us popcorn but I said no thank you for I knew I'd choke if I tried to swallow anything. We found seats and pretty soon the lights went out and there I was sitting next to James in the dark.

The movie was a western, and it soon became absorbing. There were robbers who held up a stage coach and a beautiful girl they kidnapped. There was a tall, good-looking sheriff who swung onto his horse from a running start and chased the robbers all through the picture. In the end, he saved the girl and she rode back to town on the sheriff's horse with his arms around her.

I looked over at Eunice; she was all curled up in Kenny's arm with her head on his shoulder.

When the movie was over, we filed out of the theater and started to walk home. Eunice and Kenny walked ahead and I could see they were holding hands. James and I just walked along. We talked about the movie for a while and then about his job and about school starting in a couple of weeks. He said he was excited about starting high school and that he wanted to go to college and study to be a lawyer. I said I thought all along that maybe he'd want to be a priest and he said he'd thought about that, too.

When we came to the park, instead of going around it, we followed Eunice and Kenny up the path, past the pool and up to the top of the hill. I had never been there at night and it was beautiful, but a little scary, too. The sky was black and full of stars and the trees were dark silent shapes. There wasn't a sound except the squeaking our shoes made in the damp grass. We found some big rocks to sit on and for a while we talked about the night. And then it seemed there was nothing else to talk about and Eunice leaned back into Kenny's arm and they started kissing over and over again, just kissing and giggling.

It didn't seem right to be sitting there with that going on, so I got up and started to walk down the path and James got up too.

"I'd better go home," I said.

We walked through the dark park toward the lighted street without saying much to each other. And then, it happened. Just the way I'd always dreamed it would. James was touching me, his fingers were on my fingers, locking each other into one fist and instead of melting into a heap, I stood frozen to the spot, all cold and shivering on an August night. I wanted to be home. I wished I was in my bed with nothing to wake up to in the morning but another summer day. I wished I'd never gone to the movies, or met Eunice, or ever seen James as anything except an altar boy. And, as if I needed anything else to make me completely miserable, James *kissed* me! Right there where I stood frozen to the spot, I felt his head come close to mine and the thin line where his lips came together were pressing against mine. And the only thing I felt was cold.

Eunice went back to New York and we promised we'd write to each other but we didn't. Mrs Miller went to the hospital late one night and a week later she came home with a tiny baby boy. She never did look again like she looked in that wedding picture, though.

And James, well, I guess he went to high school, for I didn't see him after school started. I didn't walk by his house any more and on Sundays I went to a different Mass just so I wouldn't see him on the altar. I began to think about becoming a nun, for there was one thing I had learned for sure - that being in love was not for me, nor getting married, nor having babies.

I was eleven that summer.

~ Split Ends ~

"There isn't going to be any baby," she said.

"What are you saying?"

They were dining at Armand's, a favorite restaurant on the upper east side, a place they saved for special occasions. Tonight they were celebrating Clint's promotion.

"I saw the doctor today," she said. "He called it a *missed abortion*."

"A what?"

"*Missed* abortion," she repeated.

"What is that?"

Marilyn, poking the fork at the food on her plate and avoiding his eyes lest she cry, said simply,

"The baby died."

"What are you talking about?"

To Clint, babies were women's work. He had opted not to join in the pre-natal exercises. He set down his knife and fork and looked at her.

"Maybe you should get another opinion," he said.

She nodded. "There was no heartbeat."

She raised her eyes and he saw that she was near tears.

"Hey, Babe, I'm sorry," he said, reaching to

touch her hand which, in anticipation, she withdrew.

"Clint, I feel rotten about this," she said.

"Hey, Babe, the kid's mine, too, you know."

She dabbed at her eyes, then looked for empathy in his.

"It would help if we could feel rotten together," she said. "Clint, we both really wanted this baby, didn't we?"

"Of course we did," he said, smiling reassurance to her. "Look, it's not the end of the world. Who says we can't have another baby?"

She looked down at the swelling of her body, gently passing her hand over it.

"I never expected anything like this," she said. "Clint, I was really looking forward to our celebration tonight."

Grateful for the change of subject, he lifted his wine glass in toast.

"Here's to the good things," he said.

She raised her glass and they clinked.

"I really wanted to celebrate," she said. "I'm very happy about your promotion."

Clint had just made vice president, his reward for exceptional management of the Palmer Hair Care account.

"Yeah," he said. "Things are really looking great. The client's happy, the boss is super happy. Babe, I'm on my way . . ."

And, realizing he'd left her concern dangling, he said,

"So, what happens next?"

"Nothing," she said. "It'll be like a miscarriage. I'll go into the hospital for a D&C and then it'll be over."

"My god!"

"It happens," she said. She wished she could sense some compassion from his response, but instead, she inferred that the whole unpleasantness was simply an inconvenience to him.

She barely touched her dinner, but she noticed that he had eaten his and when the waiter asked about dessert, he ordered chocolate mousse and *Grand Marnier*. They were silent through dessert and she didn't touch the brandy. Finally, she spoke,

"Clint, are you thinking that we needn't have gotten married after all?"

"Of course not," he protested, avoiding her eyes.

"Then why didn't we get married *before* I was pregnant?"

He shrugged.

"Then you admit the baby was the reason?"

"It wasn't *the* reason," he said.

"But now, there is no baby and you're married again - which you didn't want to be."

Abruptly, he summoned the waiter and asked for the check.

"You're too upset to talk about it now," he said.

The waiter held the chair while she got up. She followed Clint out of the restaurant. As they waited for a cab, he softened, put his arm around her shoulder.

"It's all right, Babe," he said. "Everything will work out. You'll see, life goes on."

She called her parents and Clint's to tell them her unhappy news. At work, she confided to a few. Amid a mixture of sympathy and fascination, family and friends offered comfort and support. At home, though, she and Clint rarely referred to it. For weeks, she lived in a state of anticipation, sensitive to any unfamiliar pang, never knowing when *it* would happen.

Clint's new position turned out to be more absorbing than the previous one. He sometimes brought work home, but more often, he stayed late at the office. When they were together, they talked about the burden of his work, the office politics, his deadlines, his standards and goals, his personal aspirations. He seemed to have forgotten about the baby.

Maternity clothes had been quietly bundled away in the closet with the few baby things she'd begun to collect. They had purchased no baby furnishings and the guest room had never graduated to a nursery. They went to work each morning, occasionally had dinner together and on weekends, if Clint wasn't bogged down with some project or other, they might see a show or have friends in. Life, as Clint had predicted, was going on.

It happened in the middle of the night. She woke Clint, gently shaking his shoulder.

"I have to go to the hospital," she said.

"What time is it?"

"I don't know."

He got out of bed, pulled on his slacks and a sweatshirt, slipped into socks and shoes, without a word. Finally, as they were going out the door, he took her arm.

"You okay?" he asked.

At the hospital, they answered questions: yes, she had insurance. Doctor's name? Bradley, and, yes, he had been called. A nurse came, put her into a wheel chair and told Clint he might as well go home. He leaned over the wheelchair and kissed her lightly on the forehead.

"See you tomorrow," he called as he strode off down the corridor, as though he'd just put her into a cab. Waiting for the elevator, she watched him disappear out the door.

The clock over the nurses' station said 3:25. Was this the maternity floor? Except for the two nurses on night duty, all was quiet. They wheeled her to a private room and flicked on a light, all the while chattering about something that didn't relate to her. Then, one of the nurses left and the other one gave her a gown.

"Try to get some sleep," she said. "Your doctor will see you in the morning."

"Not till morning?"

"Are you in pain?" the nurse asked.

"No," she said. "I'm just . . ."

She wasn't sure what she was - scared, lonely, sad, drained, disillusioned, hopeless - a combination of all.

"I'm okay," she said.

Alone in the quiet room and far from sleep, she waited. For mornng. For the doctor. For release from the anxiety of not knowing what to expect. She waited for Clint.

She had moved in with him two years ago when they realized they had a relationship. It had been a radical move but she had fallen in love with Clint and she was ready for any commitment. She had hoped for marriage, but Clint, having been briefly married before, was reluctant to marry again.

"Besides," he'd reasoned, "a legal document just puts stress on a relationship. You begin to count and demand and become possessive and you lose sight of why you got together in the first place."

Why they had gotten together in the first place, she thought, was because they wanted to *be* together, to share a life. According to Clint, the sanctions of church and state weren't relevant. It had made sense to her then. She had confidence in Clint's judgment, respected his decisions. She loved him, even though she sometimes doubted that he loved her as much. Whenever such doubts arose, she changed channels in her mind, flicked to stills of their lovemaking, to quiet walks together along the beach at Montauk, to intimate dinners at Armand's.

She'd met Clint at a party in Greenwich Village, an artists-and-writers gathering she'd attended with one of the designers from the office. Clint was then an aspiring writer, working on a novel. She noticed him for his wit, his charming insolence, his blatant shabbiness and she was impressed with his apparent popularity. He barely noticed her at all. Six months later, she discovered him in the Creative Department of the advertising agency where she was executive assistant to the president. Clint had been hired as a copywriter.

"Aren't you Clinton Jennings, the novelist?" she asked him.

His reaction was a mix of pleasure at being recognized and embarrassment at being discovered out of context.

"Have me met?" he asked.

45

"At a party in the Village, some months ago," she replied.

"Ah, yes, you're . . ."

"Marilyn Owens. I was there with Hal."

"Sure, I remember," he said. "So, we have a mutual friend. Great guy, Hal. He put me in touch with this job."

"But what about your novel?" she asked. "Did you finish it?"

"Oh, that," he said, dismissing it. "Somehow, you never seem to finish a first novel. Meanwhile, you have to pay the rent. So, here I am, writing copy for the rent. You work here, too?"

"Sort of," she said. "I'm George Gilroy's assistant."

"Hmm ... Cool," he observed.

They started dating, discreetly, of course, to avoid office gossip. Clint was producing good copy, had good ideas. His bosses liked him. He had toned down his insolence, shortened his hair and wore pressed pants. He was adapting to the corporate image; he had ambition.

"I could become a partner some day," he confided to her. "If I don't make any mistakes."

It would be a mistake to be caught playing with the president's assistant. But a live-together situation was imminent. There was an instability about their relationship which Marilyn felt could be cured by moving in with Clint. He liked the idea, but it had to be in secret lest they jeopardize his ambitions with the company. She agreed and for months, they lived the lie, avoiding each other at work and appearing to have lost interest in each other as dates. Eventually, though, their secret leaked, and when the gossip reached the top, George Gilroy confronted her.

"Marilyn," he asked, "is there any truth to the rumor that you and Clint Jennings are living together?"

Reluctantly, she admitted it.

"Is there any reason you and Clint can't be married?" he pried. "It can't be very comfortable living a secret life, can it?"

"It's not a secret life, George, it's my *private* life."

"I see," he said, "you're saying it's none of my business."

Silently, she concurred.

"Well, it is kind of my business, Marilyn," he said, but kindly. "We think very highly of Clint. He has talent. Clients like his ideas. He has personality. We'd like to bring him along. Believe it or not, even in this day and age - well, it's not a proper image for what we have in mind for Clint."

She looked into the face of the man with whom she had worked for six years. She knew his business. She knew his wife and their children. She had been his confidante, had taken the blame for his mistakes, had covered for him. She had always been a benevolent buffer between him and the middle management, often solving problems before they reached his desk. Now, she looked into his face with its paternal smile, the eyes unflinching and she felt as though she didn't know him at all. *It's about Clint*, she thought, *not about me.*

"This is my life, George," she said. "What are you suggesting?"

"Only this, Marilyn. Why don't you and Clint talk it over together. I'm sure something can be worked out."

"And if it can't?"

He leaned forward and smiled patronizingly. "Talk it over with Clint," he said.

They did talk it over, she and Clint, but there were no surprises. With an eye on his career, he saw a simple solution to the problem.

"Maybe we should split, Babe," he said. "I don't mean not see each other - just, you know, live apart."

"Or," Marilyn said, "we could get married."

Clint shook his head. He took her into his arms and kissed her hair, her forehead, her nose. She responded to his tepid show of fondness by wrapping her arms around him. He gently removed her, still holding her hands.

"Nothing personal, sweetheart," he said. "I'd be an ogre of a husband anyway."

"Being a husband, Clint, might be good for your corporate image."

"Now, that's a thought!" he said, with mock enthusiasm, then becoming serious. "Look, Babe, I've got plans. I'm on the way up. In another year or two, I could be on top, write my own ticket. *Then,* maybe we can think about marriage. We ought to be sure about something *so permanent.*"

She knew what he was implying, that his first attempt at marriage had not been permanent.

"*I'm* sure," she said. "I thought you were, too."

"Look, Babe, it doesn't mean we'll stop seeing each other. We'll just *live* apart."

"Or, we could get married," she said again.

They hugged, they kissed, they made love. And,

like magic, it all made sense to her again. Clint's career was foremost. He wanted success so bad because he knew he could get it. It was faster, surer than writing a novel. And when good things happened for Clint, they happened for her. Although it cost her hours, days and weeks of his attention during his period of attainment, whenever he triumphed, there was celebration. And whatever doubts she may have had evaporated in the new demonstration of his love. She was integral to his success, she knew it. He needed her applause; she was the parent to whom he showed his gold stars. And he rewarded her with an outburst of passionate love-making which was the ultimate expression, the culmination of his joy. So grateful was she that she never questioned whether his love was for her or for some intangible, an idea, a goal, a trophy . . .

Morning came. Nurses came. Doctor Bradley came. And just before they wheeled her off to the OR, Clint phoned.

"How's it going?" he asked. He was at work.
"I phoned the doctor. He explained it all to me. Said there was no point in my being there. He said you'd be fine, though. You okay?"

"I'm okay," she said.

"Everyone says Hi, hang in there," he said.
"Gilroy says hurry back, he can't do without you."

"Okay," she said again. "Clint . . ."

"Yeah, Babe?"

"Love you . . ."

"Me, too," he whispered. "See you later."

On the day she was sure she was pregnant, they

were dining at Armand's, celebrating the acquisition of a lucrative new account, the Chicago-based Palmer Hair Care Products. Clint's creative presentation had won the account and his stock, like his spirits, was high. She listened to his animated narration of how the account was won and the plaudits he had earned.

"It's happening," he said, full of excitement. "Who would have thought I'd be traveling to the top on split ends!"

"Split ends?"

"Hair care, Babe," he said. "You know, curing split ends and all that . . ."

She smiled.

"You don't *cure* split ends," she said. "You cut them off."

"Whatever," he said, raising his wine glass. "Whatever it takes . . ."

She considered postponing her announcement rather than intrude upon his excitement, but by dessert she felt she could suppress her news no longer.

"Clint," she said, "I'm pregnant."

They were married quietly, eloping over a long weekend and surprising everyone at the office with the news on a Monday morning. They made phone calls to out-of-town parents and promised to visit soon. They found a larger apartment, uptown, with a second bedroom and a much higher rent and everyone, even Clint, seemed content. And when, a month later, she revealed she was pregnant, no one was surprised.

"You did the right thing," George Gilroy said to her. "I mean making a family man of Clint."

"We did that together," she said with just a

touch of sarcasm.

Gilroy laughed.

"What I meant was that you and Clint worked it out. Everyone's happy for you. I must admit, though, I'll regret losing a good assistant."

"How come? Do you plan to fire me?"

"Of course not," he said. "I just assumed you'd want to quit after the baby comes. At least Clint thought . . ."

"Clint discussed it with you?"

"Only in passing. I assumed . . ."

"George," she interrupted. "You think I became pregnant all by myself - to snare Clint? And you think it's noble of Clint to do the right thing by marrying me? Is that what you and Clint have discussed in passing?"

Defensively, Gilroy shifted into a supervisory mode.

"Marilyn," he said, reproaching her, "suffice to say that things look very good for you and Clint. We have big plans for him. Accept that and enjoy it. And if you want to go on working, that's fine with me if you can handle it."

He looked at his watch, signalling the end of the conversation.

"I have a meeting," he said.

Instead of being burdened by marriage, as Clint had feared, it was as though he'd been liberated by it. The marriage was like a toy he'd given Marilyn to keep her happy while he nourished his career. When they were together, he was loving, passionate, attentive; at work, he was cheerful, dedicated, ambitious.

Then, on the day of his big promotion, the baby

had stopped growing.

Following the D&C, she awoke in the hospital room to see a large basket of spring flowers with best wishes from the office. She heard the phone ringing and then someone saying, "Mrs Jennings, it's your husband."

"Hello."

"Hi, Babe. Everything okay?"

"I guess so."

"It's all over?"

"It's all over."

"Great. I'll pick you up this afternoon. And, Babe," he said, "have I got good news to tell you."

As promised, he appeared, glowing with his good news, to take her home.

"It's definitely an Armand's celebration," he said, "that is, if you're up to it, Babe."

"I wish you wouldn't call me that."

"What? Babe? It's a term of endearment."

"I don't like it."

"Okay," he shrugged. "What'll it be? Honey? Sweetheart? Dahling?"

"Marilyn will do," she said, not amused. "So, what's your news, Clint? Another promotion?"

"A biggie!" he said. "Listen to this . . . Gilroy wants to open a Chicago office with me as executive vice president. He feels we should be in Palmer's town to service them like an arm of their business. It's perfect. Cuts down on the traveling. I'll be right there, on the scene. Babe - er, honey, I own this account! It's my ticket to the moon!"

Marilyn listened, hearing between the lines some

considerations that Clint's excitement was obscuring: leave New York. Find a new position in Chicago. And yet, as Clint talked about it, she didn't seem to be a part of it. She began to chuckle.

"Split ends," she said.

"What?"

"Split ends. To the moon on split ends."

"I thought you'd be happy for me."

"For you? Of course," she said, "but what about my job?"

He shrugged.

"You have options," he said simply. "You can stay on here, or you quit and come to Chicago with me."

"And you don't particularly care which choice I make, do you?"

"Of course I do," he said, taking her into his arms and planting a kiss on her forehead.

"Of course I want you with me. All I meant was that *you* get to choose what you want to do. Come on, Sweetheart, this is a celebration . . ."

She gently freed herself from his embrace. *What's to celebrate about split ends?* She wondered.

It seemed, to Marilyn, diabolical the dilemma Clint and George Gilroy had created for her. Clint, her husband of less than a year, was prepared to pick up and take off to another part of the country whether or not she was coming with him. She wished he would *insist* that she go with him, claiming her as his wife and needing her. She would go willingly. But she knew he would go to Chicago, with or without her, and leaving her behind, she felt, would not be too traumatic to him at all. Did she want to go with him? Or stay behind in the position she'd held happily for six years? She had considered it a career, confident that she did her job well, that she was appreciated and confident that, as the agency grew, so would her value to it.

Falling in love was a detour that put her on a strange highway.   Loving someone so much that children are born, suddenly noticing babies in strollers or in their mothers' arms, seeing herself in the paintings of Mary Cassatt - all of this was new to her, and Clint was the unwitting author of the fantasy. And now, it seemed that the two men in her life had conspired to dissect her life, that in this little *ménage à trois*, she was the one that mattered least.

Almost immediately, Clint was sent to set up the agency's new office in Chicago. There was much to do, staff to be interviewed and hired, offices to be established, equipment and furnishings to be bought, meetings to attend, integration with the client's business. For the first few weeks, he was a commuter, flying back and forth on the weekends, weekends they shared with his laptop. They dined at Armand's, drank *Grand Marnier*, made love, made plans. When the office was settled, Marilyn would quit her job and fly to Chicago. Then, together, they would find the ideal apartment.   With her experience, her talent for management, she should have no trouble finding the right situation.   Or, if she chose, she could do something else. Clint's executive salary was more than enough to support a trendy, social lifestyle. She needn't work at all, if she didn't want to. She could stay home and raise a family.

Then, the commuting stopped, had become too

stressful, but they talked on the phone every day. Most days. And Marilyn began to hear in Clint's voice a crisp, executive quality as he rattled on about share of market, focus groups and P&Ls, and about his excellent, hand-picked staff.

"Have you hired a secretary yet?" she asked him, cutting through the facade.

"I've got a great gal," he said, lowering his voice into the phone. "She's graying, middle-aged and a spinster."

"Why don't I come out for a weekend," she said. "We could start looking for an apartment."

"Good idea," he said. "Not this weekend, though. There's a convention I have to attend. Next weekend?"

He showed her the office, introduced her to his staff, one of which was an attractive copywriter with Cleopatra bangs and a pleasing bottom that fit firmly into her jeans. The secretary, she observed, was no older than she, had no gray hair and wore a short skirt that revealed great legs. As the boss's wife and the president's assistant, Marilyn was greeted royally, so why did she feel like an intruder? Clint had entered into a passionate love affair with his new situation.

"Babe," he said, as they dined overlooking the lake, "It's happening!"

But they didn't look for an apartment and they made love only once and Clint was either filled with nervous excitement or preoccupied, waiting for Monday morning. When Marilyn got to her own office on Monday, there was an email from Clint:

"Good morning, Babe. Great weekend," it said.

Yes, she could leave her job behind, become a dependent wife, raise babies in the suburbs, if that's what Clint wanted. But did he? He had already said he'd be an ogre of a husband. What kind of father would he be? Would this new life be, in fact, a split, with Marilyn distancing from the world in which Clint functioned and he never entering the domestic scene she'd be creating? How long would it be before Ms Great Legs, the secretary, became indispensible to Clint in more ways than one? At what point would Marilyn itch to be shuffling papers in an office again instead of piling groceries into a shopping cart?

"I think you've made the right decision," Gilroy said. Marilyn had just given him notice. "Of course, I don't know how I'll get along without you."

Marilyn smiled.

"You will, but thanks."

"Still, it's not as though you're leaving the family," he said. "I think you'll like Chicago. Clint loves it. Together you'll have a good life."

"Hmm," she said. "Well, George, I'm not going to Chicago."

"What do you mean?"

"I'm not going to Chicago. With Clint."

"But you just told me you were resigning . . ."

"Yes, George. I'm leaving my job. And I'm leaving Clint. I love you both but I need to distance from you. For a while anyway."

"I don't understand at all," George said. "What will you do instead?"

"I'm not sure," she said. "Maybe I'll go on a dig in the Andes. Or take up underwater photography in the Caribbean. Write a book. Or, who knows? Maybe start my own agency."

Gilroy laughed.

"Seriously, Marilyn," he said. "What's the matter?"

"You laugh, George? Don't you think I can do any of those things?" She paused. "Well, seriously, George, I'd like to find out what else I can do besides be a support system for a boss or a husband."

"Look, Marilyn, whatever your spat with Clint is, I'm sure it can be worked out. Meanwhile, stay on here until the dust settles and you both see things more clearly."

Marilyn sighed.

"George, this is about me. Before Clint, I was focused on you and my job. After Clint, I was focused on him. But none of us was ever focused on me. I shouldn't have to give up *me* in order to be either a good assistant or a good wife. Maybe the real me is neither of those."

Gilroy shook his head, impatient to be finished with the meeting.

"People fall in love, they get married, they raise a family," he said. "What more is there?"

"I don't know yet," she said.

"Well, there'll always be a place for you here. Have you told Clint?"

She smiled.

"Should I send him an email? He's coming next week. We'll go to Armand's to celebrate his latest triumph. He'll tell me he's had no time to look for an apartment. He'll probably bring a present that his secretary has picked out. We'll drink a lot of wine to keep the tension down." She paused. "And then, I'll tell him."

She knew he was home before she heard his key in the lock. She was ready, dressed for dinner in a simple black jacket dress, wearing the pearl earrings he'd given her for her birthday. *Pearls are for tears*; she recalled the old wives' tale. She appraised herself in the full-length mirror: her hair, softly un-styled, fell loose and playfully at her shoulders. The way Clint liked it. *Next week*, she thought, *I'll get it cut.* But tonight was for Clint. He was coming home and they hadn't seen each other in two weeks.

He let himself into the apartment.

"Hey, Babe," he called.

Her heart leapt as it always did when Clint was near, but she steadied herself and went to greet him. There he stood, handsome, virile, confident, the successful man, Prince Charming with his arms outstretched to meet her.

"Babe, you look great," he said.

His arms enfolded her in the familiar embrace as he buried his face in her playful hair and then began to peel off her jacket, walking her backwards to the bedroom. There were the eager kisses and his hands seemed to be everywhere. She felt the snap of a spaghetti strap as he tugged it off her shoulder. His kisses, his hands, his scent, his passion, enveloping, claiming, pouring love all over her. What power he had! He could make her believe anything, even that he loved her. She gave herself up to the moment and when it was over, they lay quietly in each other's arms.

"I brought you something," he said. "It's in my

bag."

"Hmm."

"What time's dinner?"

"Ten."

"Great. I could eat."

He bounced off the bed and headed for the shower. She heard the water running and just before he stepped into it, he called to her,

"Babe, have I got a lot to tell you . . ."

Marilyn regarded, on the floor, the crumpled dress with the broken strap. She picked it up, folded it and laid it on the bed where, for the last time, they had made love. Although he didn't hear her, she replied,

"I've got something to tell you, too," she said.

~ *Soup* ~

He was swimming in minestrone, thick and steamy, with chunks of beef and white pasta and garbanzo beans. His arms and legs were limp, flapping through the aromatic sea that teased his appetite but couldn't be swallowed. His stomach ached for food and his mouth gulped eagerly, only to be stopped by a painfully adamant throat.

Now, he was floating. Warm, comforting waves of soup, buoying him up, washing over his face, his eyes. Through red frames, he saw the shape of a cat on the window sill. The cat screeched and was gone through a wall of shale, and he was headed right into it. If he could only move, but his body was at once weighty and weightless. Wang! His head splintered into a million pieces.

He could see by the clock it was nearly two, daylight, afternoon. Saturday. He was probably alone in the place, this ruin of a building he shared with others like himself, the free, young people with big dreams and no money. By now, they'd all have gone, a few to part-time jobs, others to suburban home bases for a good meal.

Home. His mother would know what to do. She'd make him take aspirin and somehow force the soup through his wretched throat. And he could sleep peacefully in a white room with violets on the walls instead of shale. And when he awoke, Pecan, the little brown mutt, would be licking his face. He had been twelve when the puppy came into the family. His parents had let him name the dog Pecan. They said it was an imaginative name, that it showed he was creative.

Creative. Back then it had been a plus. How had it become a minus? *Brian has a way with words*, Miss Adams, his third-grade teacher, had said, pleasing his parents. In seventh grade, Mrs Falcone announced that Brian had *latent ability*, from which his parents inferred he wasn't trying. By tenth grade, his teachers had pronounced him unreachable, and at graduation, he was the class disaster, noted most unlikely to succeed. He had been creative enough to graduate but the only things he ever learned, he'd taught himself.

Like the guitar. Learning, he felt, was not difficult if what was being taught was something you wanted to learn. In school, they complicated everything with rules. He felt he ought to be able to split an infinitive if it felt right. Nor was history for him; he was a *now* person. And math was only a series of puzzles he had no patience for. Then, there was the confinement, the demand for his attention when he wanted to be elsewhere, thinking of other things. School was the failure, not he. School was no place for a creative person.

Down the hall, the pay phone was ringing. Someone was trying to communicate, to tell someone something good, or bad, or hopeful.

This is Man-a-Day. We have a job for you!

He'd been a man for six months, since he'd turned eighteen and left home to follow the pied piper. That's the way his father had put it, meaning that he was a fool to trade an education for the music business. The *business* of music, he'd declared, was not his pursuit. It was the words and music in his head that had to be brought together, to be sung. It was more like *religion . . . I believe in music, music almighty!*

His father had shaken his head ruefully.

"I don't know," he'd said. "I once had a ukulele, but I had sense enough not to try to make a living with it. Get your degree first. You can always play the guitar."

"Fill out this application, please. High school grad? What can you do, Brian?"

"I'm a songwriter."

"We don't get many calls for songwriters. What else can you do?"

Shit jobs.

Man-a-Day had found him a job. It was one stop on the subway, a fifty-cent ride. So he walked the twenty blocks. Three days in a row, he awoke to a nagging alarm clock, climbed into frayed, faded jeans and a tee shirt, the acceptable costume for an anything-boy. It was a dull job, supervised by an old man who knew where everything ought to be but who needed help putting it there. Not a bad guy, but a boss. On the third day, it rained hard, a cold, steady pelting rain. He doused the alarm and lay there thinking of the twenty blocks he had to walk, decided it was a legitimate reason to stay home, and went back to sleep.

"Brian, you didn't show up at your job!" The woman at Man-a-Day sounded like a guidance counselor he'd had in high school.

"It was raining," he said.

"I can't tell a client that! You have a responsibility."

"It's a long walk in the rain."

"You can't take a subway?"

"Not and eat, too."

"Listen, if you don't want the job . . ."

"Yeah, I guess I do. I'll get right on it."

"Okay, I'll tell them you'll be in. Only, Brian, don't do that again or you're through."

"Right. Okay. Thanks a lot."

So he walked the twenty blocks in the rain, lifted and shifted stock, crated and uncrated supplies, ran sundry errands. Soaked and soggy, he put in his day's work. The next day, shivering with fever, he called in sick.

The pounding, he realized, was not in his head, but on the door.

"Brian, are you in there? Somebody wants you on the phone."

"Okay, okay, I'm coming."

He raised himself on one elbow, teetering there while the revolving room came into focus. When he opened the door, Ophelia was there with the dog, Shamus, who bounded past him into the room and leapt onto his bed.

"Hey, man, what's the matter with you?" Ophelia asked, following the dog inside.

"I'm sick."

It was his mother on the phone wanting him to come home for the weekend, a train ride to Glen Cove.

"I've been trying to call you all day," she said. "Are you all right? You sound terrible."

"It's just a cold."

"Dad and I can drive in and pick you up," she said.

"No, Mom, I'll be fine."

"You can't take proper care of a cold in that miserable room."

"Look, Mom, it's just a cold," he said, "one of those soup-and-sleep colds . . ."

"Where will you get soup?"

He leaned against the wall. He was weak and the cold sweat was starting in his armpits.

"This girl," he said, "she lives down the hall. She'll get it for me. Ophelia . . ."

"O-what?"

"Ophelia. She's an actress. Lives down the hall."

"Down the hall?"

"Yeah. With her dog. Sometimes I walk the dog. So, she'll get me soup."

"Brian, I still think you should come home. Do you have a fever?"

"Oh, no, nothing that bad," he lied, and to change the subject, "Mom . . ."

"Yes?"

"I may have a job."

"A job? That's great! Where? Doing what?"

"A gig, Mom," he said, "a singing job. At the Dark Ages. It's a club. Just one night. Not much money but, you know, *exposure*."

Silence. "Oh," she said. "I thought you meant

a *job*."

"Hey, Mom, don't worry. I'm okay," he said. "But listen, Mom, I've got to go now. Say Hi to Dad."

"Brian . . ."

"Yeah, Mom?"

"This club where you're going to sing, can Dad and I come to see you?"

"You don't have to do that, Mom."

"You'd rather we didn't?"

"It's not that, Mom. It's just that, well the place is kind of dingy. I don't think you'd be comfortable."

"Oh, I see," she said. "All right. Maybe some other time."

Ophelia sprawled in the only chair in his room. She was wearing a khaki jacket over a long black skirt. On her head, a floppy red felt hat partially covered her thick, dark hair.

"You're still here?"

"I'm waiting for Frank," she said. "We're going up to Connecticut."

He sat on the bed, disturbing the dog. Ophelia went on talking but he couldn't make sense of what she was saying, something about rain and a penthouse apartment, Broadway and off-off stuff, funny stuff . . .

"Do me a favor," he said. "Will you get me some soup?"

"Soup?"

"At the Italian deli," he said.

Reluctance. "I'm waiting for someone," she said. "Besides, I just came in. I don't want to go out again till Frank gets here."

"Come on, I need food," he said.

"Where's the money?"

"There's a dollar on the table."

"What if it costs more?"

"Just get a dollar's worth. It's all I've got."

She hauled herself out of the chair and took the dollar from the table.

"Soup?"

"Yeah. Minestrone. At the Italian deli."

"Come on, Shamus," she said. The dog followed her out.

His mouth was dry, his lips and eyes burned. His throat was swollen and raw. He knew he had fever, but he had no aspirin. So what? Colds always went away. Nobody died of a cold. Besides, if he was sick, he didn't have to look for a job, or go home or do anything he didn't want to do. Just sleep. Later, when the soup came, after he ate it and felt better, he'd play his guitar. And tomorrow, if it was warm enough, he'd go to the park. He'd sit on a bench and strum and then, because it was the natural thing to do, he'd sing along to his own accompaniment, some of his own songs. Strollers would stop to listen and a small crowd would gather. They'd toss change into his guitar case. One or two might even drop in a dollar bill. On a good Sunday, he might make ten dollars.

His mother had been shocked and ashamed when he told her he sang in the streets of New York. Begging, she called it. He had tried to explain . . . songs had to be sung, they had to be heard. He wasn't forcing anyone to listen. People wanted to, and when they threw down their quarters, it was the same as applause. They were appreciating . . .

"It's because they feel sorry for you," his father had said. "They think you're some kind of a nut and they pity you."

That kind of talk had a sting to it. Some day, they'd pay lots more than quarters to hear his songs. But he couldn't expect his father to believe that.

Not that his father hadn't had it rough, the war and all that, and clerking his way through college, working two jobs and breaking his ass for a master's degree. No wonder the man valued education so. And hadn't it paid off, all that ass-breaking? The education had earned him the right to experience, and the experience then taught him to compete, to choose shrewdly, to compromise without losing. And having taken all the right steps, he had arrived at the comfortable plateau he called success. His marriage had endured, or so it seemed. Everything went well. Even the boy had been planned. He had entered at the right economic moment and the programming of his future had begun almost before his christening, developing into a pattern of disciplines that somehow only gouged an ever-widening rift between them.

But why? Every need and whim had been gratified, the best clothes, the summer trips, the ten-speeds, the club, the car . . . all this for the low-low price of obeisance to the system.

"I paid *my* dues," his father would say. "I took the flack but I never took charity!"

There was something about the way his father spoke of charity. It wasn't the faith-hope-and sort of charity, but a kind of hard-edged virtue with satellite words like donation and debt and payoff. And there were other words, his father's words, that fell like hammer blows on his head. *Responsibility.* How easy it would be to lean on a pair of devoted parents! *Integrity.* The most precious ingredient in his songs. *Determination.* The hours of practice, the bleeding fingers. And being hungry.

Where was Ophelia with the soup?

Ophelia wasn't her real name. And she was an actress like he was a songwriter, neither of them making a living at it. She had come to New York from a college in the Midwest where she had majored in dramatics. She claimed a repertoire of parts from Shakespeare to Improv and she could do accents and even nude if the script called for it. But she wasn't called very often.

Ophelia had a room down the hall. Her parents still called her Barbara, but they had agreed to subsidize her for a year, after which, if she didn't succeed at acting, she could go back to college and study something else. They paid her rent and bought her the strange clothes she wore and they kept her in spending money. But Ophelia had no intention of going back to school or doing anything at all that didn't instantly appeal to her.

He had slept, now he was waking, chilled and damp with sweat. And hungry. It seemed like hours since Ophelia had taken his last buck to buy him soup. He had been tasting it in his sleep, in his dreams. Why hadn't she come back with it? Surely, she hadn't swung with his lousy dollar. She had bucks of her own, her father's bucks. A girl could take money from her folks and not feel bad. He tried not do that. Sometimes he couldn't help it; he got too hungry or too cold. But taking money from his folks felt like a put-down whether they meant it to or not. He had to show them that he really didn't value money above his time, his freedom, his creativity. Besides, accepting money from his father made him vulnerable to the parental advice, always the same. Work hard. Go to school. Prepare yourself for life. Become somebody. Invest your youth in something that would pay off when he was forty, an obscure something his father called success, that had to do with golf and cocktail parties and property, being politic and keeping a low profile. It was not to be gained pumping gas or washing dishes or running errands, the kind of jobs he could get but somehow couldn't keep.

He didn't want to *become* somebody. He *was* somebody and the people who gave him jobs didn't seem to see that. He was *Hey-Kid* or *Hey-Stupid*. And he wanted to tell them, *Hey-Man, I ain't shit!* I can play the guitar and write songs. I've got folks who care about me and I don't cheat you . . . But to convince anybody, you had to go to college. Or be rich. Or notorious. Shrewd. Guitar players, his father said, were a dime a dozen.

And so were actresses. Damn her anyway, where was she? Addlehead. Selfish. She could be in Hoboken by now, run off on a whim with somebody she met on the way to the deli, never mind that he was hungry. Careless, irresponsible, undisciplined. Characterizing his whole generation, his mother would say.

Now, there was a woman you could depend on. Probably never in her life had she done anything on impulse, or ever wished she was anything but what she was. She had been a secretary once, before he was born, though he couldn't imagine his mother being young, like the girls he knew, the girls with scrubbed, fresh faces and no makeup, who wore jeans and went bra-less. He saw his mother in her chic Bonwit Teller suit, smelling of Arpège, with rings glistening on her fingers as they typed, her lips a delicate red, cheeks pink and powdery, with a hint of green shadow around her eyes. And the hair, always the same, a neat reddish-brown halo of waves swept back from her forehead.

He thought fondly of his mother and wished he wasn't such a disappointment to her. Perhaps if he'd had a brother or a sister to share affection, he wouldn't be such an embarrassment to her. She'd have been happy if he'd gone to med school or followed his father into business or even if he'd just been a scholar. Anything, that she could have been proud of. He was sorry about that. He wanted so much to have his mother's support. As a child, he'd felt it. Now, he was uncertain when it had been withdrawn. What gross thing had he done to destroy her confidence in him? Or had his failure grown from a feeling that she'd deserted him? Which came first? How had they veered so far from each other, mother and child, so that now they couldn't even hold a conversation? He was sorry that she thought of him as a beggar in the street, a loser. He regretted the unhappiness his behavior imposed on both his parents. And, often, he was astonished at the wisdom they seemed to have. Maybe, just maybe, they were right. But he had to find out for himself.

Ophelia was back, calling to him from the street. He opened the window and leaned out. Someone was with her. The dog was leashed to the iron railing of the steps.

"Hey, Brian," she called. "Can you come down for the soup?"

Damn!

"I'll leave it on the step. And listen, Brian, do me a favor. Keep Shamus for me. Frank and I are leaving now. See you later. Okay?"

She didn't wait for his reply, only waved again as she and her friend walked away. He slammed the window shut. Damned Addlehead! Damned Frank! And damned dog, too, as it turned out, for by the time he had gotten down the three flights, the dog had chewed open the container, spilled the soup onto the sidewalk and was eagerly lapping it up. The chawed carton was all that was tangible. He kicked it.

No use kicking the dog. It was the pattern of his life. He'd chosen the impossible path. It was always going to be like that. And yet, he knew there was a way he could erase hunger forever. He needed only to stuff his few things into a duffel bag, pick up his guitar and walk out the door. He need never shiver again in his damp room, nor walk twenty blocks to a shit job. He could wear clean clothes every day and drive a car and take out girls who wore silk blouses and shaved their legs. There was a way to cancel all the unpleasantness, the bad luck, the accidents that fate had rigged. Help was out there, waiting to be summoned. But it had its price.

He untied the dog and they went up the stairs. On the floor in his room, his guitar case waited like a faithful friend. He knelt and opened it, lifting the guitar out with care. He sat down, slipped its strap over his shoulder, steadied it across his knee and began to pick. There was a song in there, somewhere.

~ *Mulroy's Kin* ~

Mulroy checked into the Desert Breeze Motel. It was the kind of place Katie would have called cheap and refused to stay in. But Katie's days of traveling with him were over these past three years, since, sadly, he'd had to put her in the nursing home. Some kind of dementia, they called it, but he couldn't take care of her anymore, with her babbling into the mirrors and not even able to dress herself. And now, when he visited her, she didn't even know who he was.

The Desert Breeze Motel suited him fine. In his day, as a cameraman, he'd traveled all over the world, stayed in everything from flea bags to castles. The Desert Breeze was only a short cab ride from the airport and he'd rather spend the money taking the kids to dinner at a good restaurant. He had an extra five hundred dollars with him, besides a cased twenty-dollar bill he kept with his plane ticket. Usually, he didn't carry that much cash. But, just in case he found that Marilou wasn't as well off as her mother had claimed she was, he could leave her a couple hundred.

He'd been to Phoenix before, on shoots for the Army. He'd shaken hands with generals; and when they had launched Gemini into space, he was aboard the *USS Wasp* shooting pictures of the space ship's splashdown in the Atlantic Ocean. Stories like these, he felt, would make him seem more interesting to the kids than just the old codger of a relative that he was. He could tell them about man-eating fish, piranha he'd seen in the Amazon waters of Brazil, and about the movie he shot in Thailand for the missionary fathers; how he and Katie, before she got sick, had traveled all over Europe.

Of course, the kids were not kids anymore. Last time he saw Marilou, she must've been ten. She was probably nineteen or so now. The fellow, Ken, was supposed to be her husband, but Mulroy doubted that. He might be an old fogey but he knew about shacking-up. He could handle that. The main thing was getting to see Marilou before he was too old or too sick or before he died without letting her know she was to inherit his estate.

Not that he had much to leave. He'd always been a frugal man, careful with his money, but he had held onto some AT&T stock. And there was the house back east, the home he'd lived in all his life, and a nice piece of property fronting the lake. Even though the cost of Katie's illness had eaten into his nest egg, there'd still be something when he was gone, even if it was only the property. And it had to be left to someone.

He and Katie had had no children of their own. Marilou wasn't kin of his and not blood-kin to his wife, either. She was the adopted daughter of Katie's sister, Bess. He remembered the girl as a snippy kid with a sassy mouth and the sort of bad manners he wouldn't have put up with if he'd been her parent, adopted or not. But Mulroy had always had a strong urge for family. He'd lost both his parents before he was twenty, and without siblings, all the family he had were

Katie's relatives.   He'd kept in touch with Katie's widowed sister, Bess, even after Katie no longer knew who she was. A month ago, he attended Bess's funeral and it had struck him as odd that Marilou hadn't even bothered to come east to see her mother laid to rest. He hoped there was a good reason; if she hadn't the fare, he would have sent it to her. But if the girl had been hurting for money, Bess never let on to him. She always made it seem that Marilou was on top of the world, doing well and living in a fine hacienda out west. He felt that getting in touch with the girl was the least he could do for poor Bess and for Katie, even though Katie no longer knew who Marilou was or cared that her sister, Bess, had died.

Locating Marilou hadn't been easy. He'd found several phone numbers among Bess's things, no address. After he'd called all the numbers, he finally reached her. She said she was sorry she'd been unable to go east for her mother's funeral. When he called her this time, she was surprised and, he thought, not terribly thrilled, when he said he wanted to come and visit her, and she'd suggested he stay at a motel since they hadn't a spare room.

He signed the registrar's card with a proud, honest scrawl, Timothy J Mulroy. In his room, he showered and changed into his dress clothes, a brown tweed jacket over a red plaid shirt, no tie; he didn't own one. Looking into the mirror, he wondered if Marilou would remember him. She'd recognize his bald head with the salt-and-pepper fringe from ear to ear, the moustache that wrapped around the corners of his mouth and joined a cropped sandy beard that just covered his chin. He was a little stockier now and walked with a bit of a limp because of the arthritis in his hip. At any rate, she'd probably look a lot more different to him than he would to her.

He'd found a picture of her among Bess's things, a snapshot taken with this fellow, Ken. That's how she'd announced her elopement. She was pretty enough, smiling out of the picture like a model, with one arm wrapped around her fellow and his arm wrapped around her. Well, he hoped she was happy, and although it had saddened her mother that the girl had moved so far away, Bess had been consoled that at least someone was looking after Marilou.

They were picking him up at seven and he was taking them to dinner. Some place nice, he'd told Marilou when he called, and not to worry about the cost.

They were a half-hour late, which made Mulroy edgy. He prided himself on never having been late for anything in his life. Tardiness, he read as irresponsibility. But the later it got, the more worried he became that something had happened to them; or was it just that they weren't coming at all?

When, finally, he opened the door to them, he was surprised to see how tall Marilou had grown.

"Uncle Tim!" she beamed and she had to bend down to brush her lips against his cheek.

"Come in, come in," he greeted them and the girl, followed by a fellow in dungarees and a leather jacket, came in.

"This is Ken," she said and the young man, with his hands in his pockets, offered a thin smile and a nod of his head. His hair was long and a strand of it hung over one eye. Mulroy extended his hand for a shake, but Ken kept his hands in his pockets. There was no apology for being late.

"We had to borrow a car," said Marilou. "We only have a motorcycle," and she added with a nervous giggle, "We couldn't take you to dinner on that."

"Well," said Mulroy, "I hope you've picked us a good place to eat. I'm starved." What he really meant was that he'd be more comfortable with these two after he'd downed a belt of whiskey.

"We even made reservations," said Marilou. Her dark hair was drawn back from her face, making it look long and thin and she wore no makeup. When she smiled, her teeth protruded slightly. Large plastic rings dangled from her ears and the colorful long skirt and the peasant blouse that slipped over her somewhat bony shoulders gave her a costumed look.

The restaurant they'd selected was more a tavern, but if that's what they liked, it was all right with Mulroy. The fellow, Ken, didn't have much to say until they were seated and drinks had been ordered.

"So, you're a photographer," he said after he'd drunk half a mug of beer.

"Cameraman," said Mulroy. "Motion pictures - you know, movies, commercials . . ."

"Yeah? Big stuff," said Ken with a touch of sarcasm. "No weddings and bar mitzvahs?"

Mulroy could have retorted to that but he wanted no unpleasantness. He decided, instead, to turn the conversation to Ken.

"What's your line of work, son?" he asked, genially.

"I'm a writer," Ken replied, "a *creative* writer."

Mulroy translated that to mean that the man didn't have a job and he doubted Bess's fantasy about her daughter's security. Marilou was sipping a glass of white wine. He turned his attention to her.

"And you, Marilou, are you a writer, too?" he asked.

"I write some," she said, "mostly poetry."

"Well, now, there's something I don't know much about," said Mulroy. He summoned the waiter to bring another round.

"It's none of my business," he said, "but can a fella make a living writing poetry?"

"Hardly," Marilou admitted. "I also work as a waitress. I have good hours and it pays the rent."

"Nothing wrong with that," Mulroy said. He sipped his whiskey and chased it with a swallow of water.

"I guess you got lucky," Ken charged at him. "Taking pictures. You must've made some bucks in your day."

Mulroy considered Ken's remarks in poor taste, but he wasn't one to reply in kind. Besides, he hadn't come all the way across the country to fight with a disgruntled writer. He leaned across the table and looked squarely into Ken's face.

"I worked my butt off, son," he said. "I learned my craft and I made a living."

Marilou, sensing the tension, changed the subject.

"Tell me, Uncle Tim," she asked, "How's Aunt Katie doing?"

Mulroy had no wish to discuss his wife with

them.

"Katie's the same," he said.

They ate Mexican food which caused him heartburn and, afterwards, Marilou ordered margaritas. He said the salt around the glass made him thirsty, so he ordered a pitcher of beer. He hadn't gotten around to telling Marilou of her place in his will. Mostly, the conversation had been between the two of them, cryptic remarks that excluded him, with an occasional condescending nod. Something told him that they wouldn't be at all interested in hearing about his adventures. Once, he tried to talk to Marilou about her mother.

"Too bad you couldn't make it to your mother's funeral," he said, without meaning to be critical.

"I work," she said. "Couldn't get the time off."

"What kind of boss wouldn't give you time off for your mother's funeral?" Mulroy asked.

Marilou and Ken exchanged smirky looks and Ken said, "She already used the mother's-funeral excuse."

Mulroy looked from one to the other for an explanation. Marilou spoke.

"We had this good deal, an apartment in Vegas, rent-free, for a long weekend. I knew I couldn't get the time off unless it was an emergency, so I told the boss my mother died."

Mulroy stared at her, incredulous. She patted his hand.

"It's not as though we were all that close, Uncle Tim," she said. "Sometimes we didn't get along too well. And besides," she added, "it isn't as if she was my *real* mother."

"She raised you!" he cried. "Who the hell *was* your mother if not her?"

There was a band playing and people were hopping around a dance floor to a Mexican beat. Marilou and Ken got up to join them. Mulroy ordered another pitcher of beer and watched them whirling around the dance floor. The loud, twangy music offended his ears. Suddenly, he'd had enough of beer, he needed some whiskey to settle his stomach. He got up from the table and made his way to the bar. That was better. As the bartender poured, he felt more at ease.

"I never met a barkeep I didn't like," he said, raising the glass in toast. Then he laughed heartily for the first time all evening.

He woke up the next morning in his room at the Desert Breeze Motel. His head was pounding, his gut was on fire and the bed, like a turntable, was spinning him round and round. He tried to get up but he fell back. He recognized the hangover. He'd had them before, but this was the worst. He couldn't remember anything past having a few drinks at the bar with a friendly bartender. Slowly, it all came back to him. The dinner with Marilou and Ken. They must have brought him back to the motel. He laid still for a while trying to collect himself.

He was still wearing his dress clothes, even his shoes. Someone had set his glasses on the table beside the bed. They must've opened the door, dumped him and split. At length, he got up, pulled off his jacket and staggered to the bathroom where he splashed his face with cold water. He peered into the mirror at his sorry face and tried to recall whether he had offended anyone. He'd have to call Marilou and apologize. Today, he'd try to get together with her, possibly without Ken around, and then he could attend to his mission. Besides Katie, all but dead in the nursing home, Marilou was his only family. He wanted to establish that relationship and help her if he could, and to tell her that she would inherit whatever was left of his estate.

Her phone number was in his wallet. He reached for it where he kept it in his hip pocket. It was not there. He threw back the bedding; nothing. He checked the top of the dresser, the lamp stand beside the bed, the floor. Nowhere. He unzipped his canvas bag, felt through its contents and finally emptied everything out. No wallet. From the chair where he'd flung it, he grabbed his jacket, feeling for the wallet in the pockets before he reached inside. In the breast pocket he found his plane ticket and the cased twenty-dollar bill. His wallet was in the outside pocket. The soft, worn leather, curved to the shape of his hip, felt light. He opened it. The money was gone.

Sick and humiliated, he sat on the edge of the bed trying to convince himself that he'd been rolled at the bar. But then it began to sink in. Marilou wasn't blood-kin to any of them. If she didn't think enough of her mother to attend her funeral, why should she care about an old fool like him?

He put on his glasses and fished from the wallet a folded piece of paper. He dialed the number, heard it ring twice and then a woman's voice answered.

"Marilou?"

"Who you want?" The voice responded with an accent.

"May I speak to Marilou, please," he said.

"Nobody here that name," the voice replied and Mulroy thought he heard something familiar in it.

"Is that you, Marilou?" he asked.

There was no answer, just the click of a receiver hanging up.

~ *Heroes* ~

I find myself in upstate New York, attending a convention of medical suppliers with one of my sons. I live in Texas now, retired. Three years ago I lost my wife but my two sons and I keep in touch and once in a while, when one of them travels, I tag along just for a change.

From the window of my hotel room I see a city I hardly recognize, for I have been here before. I scan the facades of old buildings and see sparkling new glass towers. The downtown streets seem crowded and the city, in spite of its progress, seems small to me now. My eye wanders over the tops of buildings, the domes and clock towers, sifting through the neon, and catches a familiar sign, just barely visible in a corner of old downtown. Spelled out in light bulbs, it reads *Crown Hotel*.

Seeing that sign brings back an incident I haven't thought of in years and a name floats up through my sleeping memory, a name I am able to recall only because I've never heard anyone before or since called Gilda.

The last time I was here was during the war. I was Private First Class Warren Kendall then, assigned to a recruitment unit. There were ten of us, including the lieutenant, three corporals and a sergeant, and we were stationed at the Crown Hotel, a run-down, fifth-rate, rooms-by-the-hour dump which the army had taken over and gutted to make a barracks on the third floor.

Daniels was the sergeant. Most of us enlisted men were draftees, but Daniels was regular army. He'd already been stationed in major cities all over the country, so he knew his way around. We worked together and so we hung out together, but we didn't have much else in common. Daniels was a good-looking blond athletic type whose main concern was getting lucky. I, on the other hand, was not so handsome, although the uniform helped; but maybe because I had sisters, I wasn't as ready as Daniels was to hit on any girl that walked by. Besides, my main concern was to survive the war and get an education.

Daniels said he'd met this girl at the post office and she was a *nice* girl, not the kind you picked up in bars. She'd agreed to go out with him, but he'd have to call for her at home and meet her family. It surprised me that Daniels would be bothered doing that, but Daniels was full of surprises. The catch was that Daniels didn't want to go there alone. He didn't play well as a soloist. He needed a shadow, a straight man, a supporting cast to bring off his boy-next-door act. It wasn't the first time I'd been enlisted in his little charades. My part was to hang around through the drinking and the joking and the flirting and then to disappear. But this was the first time we'd had to play his scenario in someone's parlor. I wasn't too thrilled about doing it, but in those days everyone loved a serviceman and you only had to show up to get the red-carpet treatment. I was a little homesick and I thought it might be nice to visit a family. So I went.

Her name was Gilda. I don't remember the last name, something Italian. She was seventeen and she'd just graduated from Catholic high school. When she opened the door to us, smiling shyly, all dressed up in a pink summery dress, wearing stockings and high-heeled shoes, I wanted to run. She looked to be about twelve; probably weighed no more than a hundred pounds. She had long, silky dark hair, curled and pulled up to the top of her head where it was fastened with a pink bow. Her cheeks were lightly rouged and she wore a bright red lipstick on her small mouth.

Gilda ushered us into the parlor where her family was gathered - her mother and father, a younger sister and a small boy. As we entered, her father rose and extended his hand to Daniels and then to me, as Daniels introduced us. Her mother smiled, the children smiled. Daniels and I, splendid in our U S Army uniforms, smiled back. They invited us to sit down and offered us coffee and cake and Coca Cola. Gilda's father asked where we were from. Daniels mentioned some little town in Nebraska, which surprised me because I was pretty sure his army records had him coming from Brooklyn, New York. I said I was from Detroit, which I was, and Gilda's mother had a married cousin who lived there.

We talked a little about Detroit and Daniels set his cap on the little boy's head and everybody laughed. The kid wanted to keep the cap, but Daniels explained that he mustn't lose his regulation hat or he'd be court-martialed. That got a laugh all around and then Gilda picked up her purse, threw a sweater over her shoulders and we got up to leave. Her father got up, too, said he wondered what kind of evening we'd planned and what time Gilda could be expected home. Daniels said he thought we'd just take in a movie, maybe sip a soda afterwards and we'd have Gilda home by midnight.

I know, I know. You're thinking you sure as hell wouldn't have let your little girl go out on a date with two soldiers you never saw before. But you have to understand what it was like in World War II. All of us young men were in the service. The wartime man in uniform was a hero and heroes were never evil or dangerous to people's daughters. They were your sons and brothers and neighbors. And if a man couldn't fight for his country himself, the least he could do was be supportive to those valiant boys who could. If a couple of young soldiers, lonesome and far from home, could enjoy the company of a decent young girl for an evening on their way to war, what was the harm? It was a patriotic duty to be nice to the boys. You see, we were all heroes.

So, off we went with pretty little Gilda, but not to the movies. We started walking and Daniels reached over and took hold of Gilda's hand. She didn't object. She smiled up at him as though they were high-school sweethearts. She told us she'd just gotten her first real job, in an office downtown. She said she was an excellent typist and could take shorthand faster than anyone else in her class. She worked for a collection agency where she typed form letters to people, threatening them with lawsuits if they didn't pay their delinquent doctor bills. She didn't plan to make a career in that kind of business, but it was a job, she said, and typing is typing no matter what you're typing.

Gilda thought it was fascinating that Daniels was a *real* soldier rather than a draftee. Although she hastened to assure me that no offense was intended. She thought it was very manly, very brave for a boy to devote himself to the service of his country. Daniels thrived on her flattery and he seemed to grow taller and broader in the chest with each of her fluttery bouquets.

Before we knew it, we were only a few blocks from the Crown Hotel and Daniels suddenly had a great idea. How would Gilda like to see the barracks, a genuine barracks where the soldiers lived? I thought he was kidding, of course; he wouldn't have the nerve to take a girl into the barracks. Gilda thought it would be great fun. I suggested to Daniels that he consider the risk he'd be taking if he got caught, but I suspect he'd had it in mind from the beginning and nothing I said would dissuade him. He reminded me that there wouldn't be anyone there, only the PFC at the front desk. Daniels had a key to his own office, so we wouldn't have to pass the soldier on duty. We'd just have to walk up the three flights. It was a nervy thing to do, but that was Daniels: if there wasn't any risk, it wasn't any fun.

Gilda was impressed that Daniels had his own key and even more impressed when she saw his name stencilled on a sign on the desk. He told her he was the ranking officer and she bought that; she didn't know an officer from a non-com. I tagged along, hoping we'd soon be out of there before someone else showed up.

Beyond Daniels's small office was the barracks where we were living during the two months of this tour. He opened the door and led Gilda inside. There wasn't much to see, just a plain long room with a row of bunks and foot lockers along each wall. Gilda asked Daniels which one was his bed and which one was mine.

I stood in the doorway as he moved with her further into the room. This is the point where I was supposed to disappear. Instead, I hung back in the shadow of the doorway and watched until they were way down at the far end of the room. I saw Daniels bend down and kiss her lightly on the forehead. She didn't object. I turned away. But when I looked again, Daniels had the girl in his arms, kissing her hard on the mouth. I saw his hand go down on her butt, hiking the pink dress up over her stockings, exposing her underwear and her innocent flesh. Now I saw that she was struggling against him and I rushed into the barracks just as he threw her down on the nearest bunk and began to tear at the front of her dress. I heard her cry out, still trying with her little hands to push him away. By the time I got to them, he had sprawled on top of her, had forced her legs apart and was working at getting his pants unzipped. The girl was terrified and he clapped a hand over her mouth to stop her screams.

I grabbed his shoulders and yanked him off her. He flailed out at me and told me to get lost. I pushed him and he fell over the end of the bunk. The girl huddled in shock, disheveled and sobbing. Daniels glared at me from the floor and then he got up, tucking in his shirt and smoothing back his hair. I called him Buddy and put my hand on his shoulder to reassure him that the incident was history. Then he ran out and left me with Gilda.

The girl was really shaken. I supposed she was a virgin. I supposed she'd never even been kissed hard on the mouth before. I supposed also that it would take a long time before she'd want to be kissed again. I picked up her sweater and settled it around her shoulders, then I helped her to her feet and took her out of there. She didn't want to go home; she was too upset. She didn't want her family to know what had happened.

We sat in a coffee shop, neither of us saying much, except after a while she'd start to cry again. What could I tell her? Don't pick up soldiers in post offices? Or, all soldiers aren't heroes and heroes aren't always what they seem to be. I told her I was sorry about it, and she said she was glad I was there or he would have . . . she had trouble saying the word . . . she might have been *raped!*

Finally, I delivered her safely to her front door. She thanked me and we said goodbye.

The incident went swiftly from my mind. I had a war to get on with. However, Sergeant Daniels and I didn't hang out together anymore. And when our two months were up, he was sent to some place in Illinois and I wound up in Alabama. We didn't keep in touch.

During my three-year hitch, I met a lot of GIs and every once in a while I'd run into somebody who'd known Daniels. Once I heard that he'd been shot in a saloon brawl. Another time a fellow told me Daniels had shipped out and had been killed in combat somewhere in Italy. And after the war, when a bunch of us got together for a reunion, the story was that Daniels had gotten himself dishonorably discharged from the army and he'd married a farm girl in Iowa where he'd settled down to raising chickens. I suspect that was probably more a joke than a fact.

But Gilda . . . I wonder what became of her. I

wonder how long it took her to recover from that night, how long before she trusted again. Did she ever find her hero and are they out there somewhere in this city, happy together, blessed with prospering grown-up kids and beautiful grandchildren? I'd like to think so.

As for Daniels, I may never know for sure what happened to him, but I wonder how many Gildas there were in his valiant career. I prefer not to dwell on it. For me, Daniels died quite unheroically that night over there in that sorry place with the light bulbs spelling out Crown Hotel.

~ *Puppy Love* ~

A week after she met him at a party, she did a daring thing - she phoned and asked him to take her to lunch. When his secretary asked who was calling, she felt foolish answering, *Mrs Baxter* and almost hung up instead. Then, she quickly added, *Lois. Lois Baxter.* He might not remember her married name. He would surely remember Lois.

Before she phoned, she asked herself how she would feel if a childhood sweetheart phoned her husband. She was too sophisticated, she thought, to feel jealousy. After all, she and Steve had been happily married for too many years to feel insecure. Why, then was she trembling in a phone booth, losing her cool to a secretary?

She and Guy had been high-school sweethearts and when he had popped up, so inappropriately, at Helen Gibson's dinner party, he had rustled a bag of old memories and fanned a little spark which, she thought, had flickered out long ago.

By the time she reached forty-five, Lois had done everything a woman was supposed to do. She had married the man chosen by his class most likely to succeed and he had. She had borne three bright and beautiful children, become proficient in the homemaking arts and was considered an innovative hostess. She was blessed with an impressive collection of credit cards, a car of her own and a custom-built home on a wooded acre in Westchester County.

But, lately, she had come to feel that she belonged to a colony of clones who entertained each other at cocktail parties and buffet suppers; who conversed seriously about the generation gap, crime in the streets and home improvements. The women visited the same salons, shopped in the same stores, and appeared at parties in the same casual chic. Their men drank Scotch, exchanged stories and traveled a lot. They all indulged in harmless, ego-building flirtations, but were generally faithful to their spouses.

Habitually a conformist, Lois had gradually become disenchanted. To remodel herself as an individual, she looked for hobbies. She joined a class in beaded flower-making and, after she had potted everything in sight, there followed piano lessons, an adult education class in creative writing, a computer course (with an eye toward getting a job) - each venture aborted by another party, a committee, one of the children's projects or a trip with her husband. She felt like the moving part in a machine which no one noticed until it stopped functioning, and it was becoming clear to her that a moving part had no business functioning on its own. There were times when she thought of running away, without malice or fury, just going away somewhere to discover what, underneath the stylish hair, the makeup and jewelry, Lois Baxter really looked like.

Meeting Guy Markham at Helen's party was a timely interruption to the placid existence from which she wished to flee. They hadn't even recognized each other until she heard his name and then there had followed one of those stock conversations that promised to lead nowhere.

"Guy?" she had asked, tentatively, "Guy Markham from Erie whose father ran the candy store?"

After a second, when he recognized her, he exclaimed, "Lois Hills!"

They laughed together, grabbing each other's hands and holding tight.

"Imagine . . . after all these years!"

"It's a small world . . ."

"What on earth brings you here?"

Guy Markham, she learned, had been transferred from the Coast to his firm's New York office. His wife and children would follow in a few weeks. In the meantime, an office buddy, Matt Gibson, was attending to Guy's leisure hours.

"Beautiful," Matt said, "you two knowing each other. You'll have a lot to catch up on."

But they didn't catch up on anything. Helen had snatched Guy away to introduce him to other guests and they were not seated near each other at dinner. Afterwards, her husband, feeling miserable with a cold coming on, made their apologies and took her home. Later, though, he said,

"That fellow, Markham, the one you went to school with - you ought to ask him out here for a weekend. Do you think he plays golf? He'd probably appreciate getting out of that hotel room . . ."

"Yes," she said, simply. "I'll call him."

It was the obvious, friendly thing to do. But for some reason, she did not want Guy to visit her home, to play golf with her husband or to meet her children. Rather, she would erase all those years and be fifteen again, lying on a grassy hill in the Knollwood golf course, finding shapes in the great white cotton clouds that sailed over their heads, and making little electric thrills when they touched each other.

Guy had filtered out of her life as naturally as had her geometry book and her shabby jeans. The memory smelled of gardenias and was flecked with the dancing lights of a prom's crystal ball. A girl with long, brown hair, wearing perfume and pearls for the first time, perspired under the boy's urgent clasp. From time to time, he touched her forehead with his lips, not really a kiss, but saying much more. Later, they had kissed with soft, dry lips and told each other, *I love you. Oh, how I love you!*

And then it was over. That first tentative embrace had been lost, buried in youth and innocence, and the sweet, embarrassed kiss had long ago faded on her lips. Love, with its aching uncertainty, the delicious promise of the never-to-be-tasted fruit, was gone like the clouds on the hill.

But she did not recall the end. She only remembered love, pure and innocent, elusive as a dream - the uncapturable joy of untried love. How could she defile that memory? She had no wish to demonstrate to Guy how happily married she was or to prove her talent as a hostess. He would be as out of place in her home as Steve and the children would be in the memory. No, she would not call and ask him out for the weekend.

But she did call him.

They went to one of those quiet little restaurants that imitate French cuisine and take a long time serving it.

"I'm in town to do some shopping," she lied, "and I thought it would be fun to see you again. Do you mind my calling you?"

"I'm glad you did," he said. "I was disappointed we didn't have more time together at the Gibsons' party. You look great, Lois."

"Thanks, Guy. You look great, too."

It was simply banter. He looked older, of course, except when he smiled and then, with his face seeming fuller and his eyes brightened, she caught sight of the boy she remembered.

"Tell me about your family," she said when the wine had been poured.

"Well . . ." He paused to sip his wine. "Carole's my wife," he said, "and I have two boys in high school."

"Would I know Carole? Is she from home?"

"No. We met at the university." He grinned. "I'm afraid I married over my head," he said. "Carole's the brainy one in the family."

"And you're still the life of the party, I'll bet," said Lois. "Do you still play the piano?"

"Oh, yes," he said. "At parties. Still the clown."

"We had fun," she mused.

He reached into his breast pocket and took out his wallet, opening it and passing it across the table to her.

"The inevitable photos," he said.

She looked at the polished faces of his two boys and exclaimed, "So handsome!"

"They look like their mother," he said.

Lois scanned the photograph of the pretty blond woman with clear, serious eyes who was the brains of the Markham family.

"She's lovely," she said and handed back his wallet.

"Carole's a child psychologist," Guy said, and Lois felt a pang of envy at the note of pride in his voice.

"How very fortunate for your boys," she said.

He grinned.

"The shoemaker's children are not always well shod," he said.

"Now, what does that mean?" she pried, sensing some flaw in the beautiful and talented Carole.

"Nothing, really," he said. "Only that I'll bet your kids are much the same as mine. Kids are the same. We were the same. Only then we rode bicycles. Now they drive cars."

Lois remembered riding on the crossbar of Guy's bicycle and she smiled wistfully.

"It's funny," she said, "they miss a lot having so much."

"They're a whole lot smarter than we were," he said.

"In a way, that's sad . . ."

"They wouldn't think so. They know it all."

"I guess that's what I mean," she said. "It's sad when you've learned it all - when there's nothing left to discover."

He eyed her with amusement and teased, "Are you going profound on me?"

She blushed, returning her eyes to the wine.

"Private joke," she said. "It would take me twenty-five years to explain."

She raised her wine glass and finished it all too fast. He refilled her glass.

"I was really surprised when you phoned," he said. "Pleased, but surprised."

"Why surprised?"

"Because you were always so shy," he said.

"Was I really? You were the basketball hero. I was flattered to be your girl."

"You still are - shy, I mean."

"Why do you say that?"

"Because you're sitting there like a lady, behaving as though we had met for the first time. Don't you remember anything?"

He grinned, leaning toward her and placing his hand on hers.

"You were the first girl I ever wanted to make love with."

Lois began to tremble with a many-faceted pang. His eyes were bright with excitement.

"Was that - it?" she asked, feeling chilled.

"Yes."

"We - never did."

"No."

"And when you saw me at the party . . .?"

"I remembered that."

"That you wanted to sleep with me?"

"Yes."

"That's funny," she said, withdrawing her hand.

"Why is it funny? You were the prettiest girl in the school. Now, you're a beautiful woman."

She lowered her eyes.

"Was that it, Guy? Was that what I've been remembering?"

"Well, of course, that wasn't all of it . . ."

"We thought we were in love," she said. "How naive . . ."

"It's what they used to call puppy love," he said.

"I missed you all that summer. I thought I would die before I'd see you again and then in the fall, you went off to college."

"That summer," he said, "your family had a place at the lake and I had a camp counseling job. And then, yes, I went off to college."

"I remember you phoned me when you came home for Christmas. We got together but it wasn't the same. We didn't even kiss. We were like strangers."

He poured more wine.

"Things happen, they change you," he said.

"And now," she said, "here we are again - two strangers sipping wine over an old memory."

"I always wanted to make love with you," he said. "When I saw you at the party . . . I still do."

He was gazing at her with crisp anticipation and she was troubled by the frank invitation in his eyes.

"Without love, without commitment? A fling?"

He shrugged. "For old time's sake . . ."

His hand, warm and moist, found hers again and the wine sang in her veins. Somewhere near them a candle flickered and glasses were clinking against one another. They gazed at each other, suspended in a moment that would never come again, a moment in which she felt all the careless, uncluttered sweetness of an innocent love well up and overflow once more, only to be washed back again into the sea, this time forever. The man across the table pouring wine into her glass and inviting her to join him in a fling bore no resemblance to the boy in the memory and she was no longer the girl.

The waiter was standing over them.

"Are you ready to order?" he intruded.

Startled, she withdrew her hand and glanced at her watch.

"Oh, Guy," she said. "Look at the time. I've kept you far too long. And I must run."

He paid the check and followed her out of the restaurant.

"It's been wonderful seeing you again, Guy," she said, extending her hand to shake his. He leaned down and kissed her on the cheek.

"If I've offended you . . ."

"Certainly not," she said, and just before she walked away, she added, "Oh, Guy, I almost forgot . . . My husband and I would like to have you spend a weekend with us in Larchmont. Can you come? Do you play golf?"

~ *Gus* ~

I am in labor. I am having his baby and all he can think of is that he's missing an audition. I apologize, offer to take a cab to the hospital by myself. For a moment he considers it, then decides that he can still make the audition. He grumbles, says labor's supposed to start in the middle of the night, not at nine in the morning. I don't tell him that labor's been going on since four.

The baby is two weeks late, so my bag is packed and I've put away cab fare. My delivery will take place uptown in New York Hospital where, for the last seven months, I've been a clinic patient. This baby has been a complication in our lives.

We were doing all right as long as I was working, but when I began to show, I had to resign my job as receptionist. They gave me a baby shower and took up a collection and all that, but pregnancy wasn't pretty and besides, everyone knew Chaz and I weren't married.

The reason this audition is important to Chaz is that it's for a television commercial. Television. That's this new medium that some think will revolutionize the advertising business, and that a few cynics think will never get off the ground. Nobody we know owns a television set, but you can sit in a bar and watch it, or you can stand in the street and watch it through the window of an appliance store that sells sets. We've done that. Chaz is very enthusiastic about television. He says it's the future of the whole entertainment industry and he longs to get into it while it's still young. He'd even work for nothing to get his foot in the door. Chaz is good at that, working for nothing, which is why I have to squirrel away cab fare.

I begin to distinguish cramp from pain and by the time the cab makes its way through rush-hour traffic from Fourteenth Street to East Seventieth, I'm well on my way to becoming a new mother. The cab lets us off at the emergency entrance. A nurse puts me into a wheel chair and asks me questions. She writes my answers down on a form. I give her my name, Diana Johnson. She looks at Chaz and calls him Mr Johnson. He quickly sets her straight and announces himself as Chaz Boudreau. She doesn't care. She tells him that he can wait but that it will probably be several hours. I wish him good luck with his audition and he gives my forehead a kiss, promising to see me later.

I'm in the labor room. They made me take a shower. I could hardly stand up with the pain. All through the pregnancy I couldn't wait for it to begin, now I wish it would stop. It's like being on a roller coaster, terrified to be there, but you can't get off. There's another woman in here with me. Between pains, we exchange bits of conversation. Her name is Elsa and she's having her third child. She tells me her first one kept her in labor for sixteen hours. I begin to count the hours from four this morning. The clock on the wall reads a little after noon. I comfort myself that by this time tomorrow, it'll all be over.

When I first suspected that I was pregnant, I took a large dose of castor oil and hoped it would go away. Obviously, it didn't. Chaz was astonished, as though he'd never heard of pregnancy and as though he'd had nothing at all to do with it. He agreed to help, though; he'd ask around and find out how one located a doctor that did abortions. The remnants of my moral scruples leapt up like ghosts, waving little cautionary flags: *illegal, dangerous, sinful* . . . I told Chaz I'd prefer not to have an abortion and he railed at me. *What're you going to do with a kid!* Not what are *we* going to do.

Chaz had given me a weighty question to ponder. I could hardly earn a living and raise a child alongside a struggling actor in the tiny studio apartment we shared. We had indeed created an impossible situation. *There ought to be some kind of pill you could take.* That was Chaz's solution. I told him there was and it was called poison. He didn't appreciate the sarcasm and he thought it was a dumb thing to do, to get pregnant when it didn't fit in with our lifestyle. I said I'd heard about a simple operation called a vasectomy that he might like to look into. Such proposed tampering with his virility was, of course, unthinkable. That was the way our arguments went in the early weeks of *my* pregnancy.

I've been dozing, it seems like hours, between pains. Nurses come in periodically to check on the fetal heartbeat. They give me ice chips, take my temperature and pulse, speak kindly to me. They ask if I've picked out names. Suddenly, my entire body seems to erupt in one great spasm that threatens to propel that wretched creature straight through my stomach wall. I scream and, as if in response, it settles down again. I lay panting and sweating and cursing. They pat my hand and tell me it won't be long now.

When I began to show, I not only became unemployed, I also became an embarrassment to Chaz. An aspiring young actor couldn't afford to be seen about with an obviously pregnant non-wife. A wife would be bad enough, but a pregnant girlfriend would be anathema to a hopeful's career. I agreed to stay out of sight and Chaz agreed to get some kind of paying job. We were sealing our union in reciprocal cruelties. Chaz became a waiter at a Schraffts' restaurant and I kept to myself, growing our baby in secret.

Once a month, I'd take the bus up to the clinic for a check on my fitness. I never saw the same doctor twice and I was too healthy to attract special attention. About three months ago, I stopped in at the Social Services Department to talk about my dilemma. I always left the hospital feeling dejected and forlorn, sorry for myself. Chaz hated his job, but it paid our rent and, working nights, he was able to make the rounds during the day. He managed to land some work, small parts on radio shows, not much; just enough to keep up his morale. Life was almost pleasant then. We might even go to a movie and hold hands in the dark. Although we rarely discussed it, always hanging over us like a banner of truth was the question, *What're you going to do with a kid?*

I can't stand it anymore! Do something. Kill me! I am screaming and now they're all paying attention. I'm being lifted onto a gurney and wheeled away, just a short trip from the labor room to the delivery room. Thank God! I'll soon be delivered from all evil . . . My eyes flit wildly from one to another of them, these strangers talking unintelligibly through their masks. They clamp something over my nose and mouth. Now we are all masked. We are counting backwards, ten, nine, eight . . . *push!*

When I open my eyes, I am retching into a steel basin the nurse is holding. The ether has made me sick. I wonder if it is over or if I still have more to go through. Someone is saying my name. *Diana, you have a beautiful little boy.* I lie back on the flat, pillowless bed and let myself go limp. As they wheel me to the ward, they are asking me if I would like to see him, my son, and I am saying no.

I'm not going to tell you how wretched I am. You can fill that in for yourself. Imagine you've just given birth after nine interminable months and twelve hours of labor and you're exhausted. Imagine that you have no husband holding your hand, telling you how great you are and how proud he is. Imagine the women in the other beds wearing bed jackets and ribbons in their hair, surrounded by flowers arranged in ceramic baby booties and stork-shaped baskets. Imagine how you'd like to get up out of bed and get on with your life so you could turn off this faucet of self pity that keeps filling up your eyes. Imagine the scrawny little creature wrapped in a blanket and wailing away in the nursery and how you keep pushing him out of your mind.

It is visiting hours. In the bed across from me, I recognize Elsa. She'd had her baby, a girl, hours before I was even close. She waves to me and says congratulations and I am glad to see her, as though we were old friends. Later, she tells me that she's had her tubes tied so she won't get pregnant again. There are three other women in the ward and three empty beds. Only the fathers are allowed on the maternity floor. One by one they come, the husbands. A mother who is allowed out of bed, leans on her mate's arm, gingerly steps into her slippers and together they walk out to view their baby through the window of a glassed-in nursery.

I am still a little groggy and I think I see Chaz standing there. He is holding in his hand a bouquet of daisies. He looks silly and I begin to laugh. He extends the flowers to me. I try to sit up but it hurts, so I slump back down, and Chaz puts the daisies in my water glass beside the bed. He stands there looking uncomfortable, doing his duty. I ask him how the audition went. He says he thinks he got the job; at least they called him back and what's even more thrilling, he's been asked to read for a running part in a new television daytime drama series. He is full of excitement as he tells me that television is where his future lies, he feels it in his gut.

I'm not saying much, just absently listening until I hear him say, *I saw the kid.* My kid that I hadn't even seen. He shrugs it off saying that they all looked alike. He wants to know when I'm getting out of here. They keep you seven days, I tell him.

The current thinking is that formula is better than breast feeding, so none of the mothers is nursing. They bring the babies into the ward at regular times so the mothers can feed them. By mistake, they bring mine, even though I've told them not to. A nurse comes and lays this bundle in my arms, hands me a bottle. I can't help myself; I have to look. I have never seen a newborn baby before. I am afraid of it. Elsa calls over to me. "Toe-counting time," she says. She tells me to unwrap the blanket and count the fingers and toes and to check the other little digit just to be sure it's all there. She has two boys. I do as Elsa says and everything's intact. It squirms, it quivers, it cries. I rewrap the bundle and poke the nipple of the bottle into its mouth. It doesn't care about me, only that stuff in the bottle. And, as I listen to the contented murmurings of its sucking, I look into its face, seeing its half-opened eyes, the ruddy cheeks, the fringe of reddish down about its forehead and I come to terms with the fact that this peculiar little creature is my son. A name pops into my head, coming from I don't know where. I'm smiling, feeling something very warm and intense inside me. I speak to it. *Hi, Gus.* That's all I can say.

The doctor says I can go home today. I'm dressed and my bag is packed. They're shooting Chaz's commercial so he's not coming for me. I'm taking a cab. Elsa went home yesterday. She gave me her phone number and said let's keep in touch. Regretfully, I toss it into the waste basket.

The woman from Social Services was here. She explained what everybody's rights are and she brought papers for me to sign. I just want it to be over with. I sign. Now, while I'm waiting for the nurse to escort me to the lobby, I take a walk down the hall to the nursery window. I look in. He's still there. He's asleep, his perfect little fist clenched against his cheek. He doesn't realize we've spent his first week together. And it

106

doesn't matter at all to him that we'll never know each other.   I take a long, reverent last look at this remarkable little being.

I hope you have a wonderful life, I tell him through the glass. *Goodbye, Gus.*

The nurse is coming with the wheel chair.   It's time for me to leave.

~ *The First Nine Months* ~

They told me to write it down. The doctor feels that facing the reality of what I did might help to deliver me from the chaotic state I find myself in. Actually, it was JP's idea and, considering the humiliation he's suffered, I can hardly refuse to do anything he asks.

It began at Gladys Henning's baby shower. No, it really goes back further than that. I must start with JP and me and tell how we met and why he married me.

Before I finished school, I had very carefully gone over my aptitudes and sensibly concluded that I'd better find myself a husband. He must be good-looking, virile (I'd want lots of kids), intelligent, strong and, of course, I'd have to be hopelessly in love with him.

I ruled out college on the off-chance I might fall in love with a perpetual student. With an eye to snaring a rich pediatrician, I considered nursing, but I couldn't rise to the attendant blood and bedpans. I thought about becoming an airlines flight attendant. That seemed a promising exposure to a variety of attractive types - diplomats, celebrities, tycoons. But there wasn't enough time during the course of a plane flight to insinuate my better qualities. I'm no sex object who can deliver the mail with one or two well-placed undulations.

I decided I would be exactly the right wife for a

corporation executive, so I went to business school and learned to type well enough for Miss Perkins to graduate me and place me with a large midtown insurance company. I served my time in the steno pool and eventually I became a Secretary. On that happy day, I was *given* to one John Patterson Willis, a new claims manager, who was tailor-made for my marital plans.

Not only was John Patterson Willis unmarried, he was uncommonly handsome and those in the know rated him most likely to succeed in the insurance business. The next step was to get the target to aim at the arrow. I'm not exactly a plain Jane, but I'm no cover girl either. I'm too plump to be considered sexy and my features are too sharp for all-American girl. I'm not the athletic type and I'm certainly no brain. I'm just an ordinary Mrs Somebody who developed a talent for cooking to go with a weakness for eating.

No, snaring John Patterson Willis wasn't going to be easy. Being his *girl* (You can leave the message with my girl . . .), I had the drop on other contenders, but my methods of attracting his attention, involuntary as they were, were hardly likely to win the prize. For instance . . .

"Miss Burke," he'd say, with strained patience. "Mr Elroy is waiting for the Jackson file."

"Mr Elroy?"

"Lucius Newton Elroy, senior vice president of this firm."

"Oh, *that* Mr Elroy . . ."

"Miss Burke!" How exasperated he could get! "Where is the Jackson file and why isn't it on Mr Elroy's desk?"

I couldn't very well expect John Patterson Willis to understand the confusion in my shorthand notes that led me to transcribe *destroy* instead of Elroy.

My problem at that point was not so much winning a husband as it was holding my job, even though I was certain I could handle the role of wife more competently. That JP didn't demand a replacement for me, I attributed to a weakness for weak things. Or, possibly, I reminded him of a favorite aunt. Anyway, he seemed determined to sweat it out with me and I continued to limp along as *his girl.*

Then, one night, things brightened. We had been working late and JP invited me to have dinner with him, legitimately, of course, on his expense account. Away from the office, we got to know a little about each other and I inferred that he was much too busy becoming an executive to have time for screening a wife. That made me pretty nearly the most important woman in his life, except his mother, but she was living way out in Omaha. So, I decided to invite him to my place for a home-cooked dinner. I may not glow in a dim-lit cocktail lounge, but in the kitchen, I shine.

As it turned out, JP loved to eat. You'd never know it to look at him. He's tall and slim, even gaunt. But the way he took hold of a knife and fork and put them to work on my chicken and dumplings was most encouraging. The next time he came, he asked for seconds and before I knew it, he was hinting about his favorite dishes. One night he revealed that he had put on six pounds.

"I'm fattening you up for the kill," I said.

"What?"

"Nothing. Just an old farm joke."

"I didn't know you were a farm girl."

Oh, well. I wondered if he knew the one about the way to a man's heart being through his stomach. Probably not. Anyway, things were progressing nicely and we discovered we had one significant thing in common - we both like children.

"I like kids," was the way he put it.

"Me, too," I said. "I'd like a houseful."

He looked as though he'd just discovered something.

"I'll bet you'd be a great wife and mom," he said.

"Try me," I said. But JP didn't get the joke until much later on, specifically, the day he fired me.

He had been very reserved all that day and at quitting time, he called me in to his office, looking grave.

"Miss Burke - Laura," he began. He wouldn't call me by my first name around the office, although we were certainly good enough friends by now.

"I don't quite know how to tell you this," he went on. "I've just been promoted."

"That's wonderful!" I cheered.

"Thanks, but I can't take you with me. You know that at my level, the men aren't entitled to choose their own girls. I'd ask for you if it would do any good."

I said sure.

"I guess they'll want you to stay on with the man who takes my place."

I said sure again.

"I'm damned sorry, Laura." He meant it, too.

"It's okay, JP," I said, shrugging off my whole future. "Good luck upstairs."

He said thanks again and I rushed out, going

straight to my apartment where I kicked a couple of chairs and banged a few pots and pans and phrased an irate letter of resignation to the firm which was handling things all wrong. Just as I had my campaign nicely under way, they had yanked the whole project out from under me. It wasn't likely that I would look as good to JP on the seventh floor as I had on the sixth and he might decide, upon exposure to some of the firm's fancier females, that good food was not as important as some other things.

Everything came out all right, though, just as it does in the movies. In the last scene, just before I committed theoretical suicide, JP appeared at the door and said he had thought of a wonderful idea. It went something like this: he said,

"Let's get married."

I said, "This is so sudden."

He said, "Well, it just never occurred to me before."

"Are you sure you're not just being nice?"

He said, "Oh, no. I've been thinking. A man really ought to have a wife and a family. And," he added, "I've become quite fond of you."

That's how we became engaged.

I wanted to be married right away, but JP said there was no hurry, that for propriety's sake, we should do it right. I blush to think of what he meant by that, but I had to agree that the fine, stable image he'd presented so far could be damaged by something unconventional, like a hasty wedding. So we drove upstate to visit my mother and announce our plans and the next weekend we flew to Omaha to break the news to JP's family. All went well. My mother took over. She knew just how to run a wedding, having seen my two sisters elegantly launched back home.

JP and my mother felt we should be married in June, a wait of almost a year.

"How about Christmas?" I suggested.

"Ridiculous," my mother said. "The weather could be awful. Besides, people have other things to do during the holidays."

I finally won, when I pointed out to JP that he had two weeks of vacation to use up before the end of the year, so we set the date in December.

I stayed on at the office and played secretary to JP's successor, although my motives were not entirely pure. I rather enjoyed flashing JP's ring around and besides, I could keep an eye on him. After all, we weren't married yet and if I could tip him over, what would happen if someone more talented took a run at him? Towards the end of November, I gave my notice and before I left, the girls gave me a shower, complete with giggles and bawdy predictions and scads of lovely gifts.

Between my mother and JP and his mother, we came up with a guest list of a hundred and fifty, nearly all of whom attended our wedding. Ancient friends of my mother came from miles away, wrung our hands and recalled when I was just a little thing with soggy pants and a pot belly. Of my family, only my sister, Amy, in Georgia, the one with five kids, couldn't make it. Most of JP's family, sisters and brothers, cousins, aunts and uncles, came from the midwest. Even some of the firm's executives who JP felt it proper to invite, each came with a wife on his arm, each staying long enough to look us over and, I suppose, evaluate our future with the company.

We honeymooned in Bermuda and I discovered that, hidden beneath the business suit, was a real live man who tripped over his own feet after the second margarita. I saw him with his hair mussed and with sweat pouring off his face after a tennis game. I saw him yawn and I heard him snore, all of which assured me that JP was irrevocably mine. My mission was accomplished and I was at last going to function as a loving wife and breeder of little Willises. JP told me all about his childhood and revealed his plans to advance with the firm. I was a little surprised to learn how calculating he was about it, but he patted my hand and said,

"Don't worry about a thing. All you have to do is stay home and have babies."

When we returned, JP, back in his business suit, thought we should look for a house in the suburbs.

"A man ought to have his own home," he said. "It shows a sense of responsibility."

We settled on a little Cape Cod with an expansion attic. It wasn't exactly what JP had in mind. He had his fantasies, too. But I thought it was just fine.

For the first year, I played house. I took weeks to decide on drapery and months to pick out a chair. I threw myself completely into problems like whether to hang a mirror or a painting over the fireplace. I went overboard on a pair of boudoir lamps that threw no light but looked quaint on the night tables. I changed the decor of the bathroom once a week (all those shower-present towels). We entertained grandly or at the drop of a hat, and I soon got the knack of being the wife of a promising young insurance executive. Everything was fine except for one thing. A phrase kept intruding, like a nudge . . . *when the babies start to come.*

Nearly two years went by and no babies came.

"Maybe you should see a doctor about it," JP urged over coffee one morning, so I toddled off to see one. His report was discouraging.

"It's not likely I'll have any babies," I told JP with a quivering lip. He reacted to that as though I'd hit him with a ball bat.

"That's crazy," he cried, "you're a natural for kids!"

Without exactly saying so, he made me feel like a baby machine he'd invested in only to find out it didn't work.

"Maybe you can get your money back," I said.

"What?"

"Nothing." I pouted.

JP felt we should get another opinion, so I looked up a top-flight obstetrician and I put the problem to him. Dr Broadbent was thorough, he was sympathetic, but he wasn't encouraging.

"A chance in a thousand," was the best he could do. "You might consider adopting . . ."

But I wasn't ready to give up. What's more, I wasn't sure I was going to deliver this desperate news to JP at all. In fact, I wasn't going to mention it to anyone. I couldn't see putting the matter of my infertility on the chopping block to be carved up by all the experts in the business - my mother, his mother, my sisters and an assortment of in-laws and friends - everybody who ever had or never had a baby.

"You see," said JP, happy again. "That first doctor didn't know what he was talking about."

I had told him that Dr Broadbent was going to give me treatments, that he'd had cases like mine before and that after treatments the results were amazing. One woman, I said, even had triplets.

"Is that so?" JP bought the whole story.

Among our intimate friends, we discussed the situation hopefully. Everyone agreed I couldn't be in better hands than Dr Broadbent's who was tops in his field. So, every Tuesday afternoon, at exactly a quarter to two, I got into the car and drove to a mythical appointment with Dr B.

This went on for months, with everyone checking regularly to see if there was any change. JP had developed an annoying habit of scanning me from top to toe each morning to see if I'd developed any new curves and my mother called weekly for a progress report. I boxed very cagily and fended them all off, saying *Patience!* Meanwhile, I had seen every movie for miles around (I had to do something on those Tuesday afternoons) and each month, I drew a check to the order of Dr Broadbent to pay for my "treatments." Of course, Dr Broadbent never saw them, but I handled the bookkeeping, so JP didn't know that. Periodically, to make it seem real, I'd let him know how much they were costing.

"I hope they pay off soon," he muttered. Anyway, he believed they would pay off. I knew I couldn't keep it up much longer.

Now, we come to Gladys Henning's baby shower. In a way, it wasn't all my fault. I didn't want to go in the first place, but I couldn't get out of it. Well, it was awful. It was nice for Gladys, of course, but for me it was awful. There I sat among a group of women, every one of whom was either a mother or obviously expecting to be one. Except me. And, to make it worse, I had to bring them up to date on my condition because women are interested in each other's reproductive capacities and nothing delights us more than hearing about a new pregnancy. So, what I did - it just came over me to do it - I hadn't planned it, but the next thing I knew, I heard myself saying *I'm pregnant.*

"He did it! That marvelous man, he did it!" They were talking about Dr Broadbent, not JP.

Another little lie. I could handle it. In a few weeks, I would tell them that it was a mistake. Funny how one little lie begets a bigger one.

A few days later, JP phoned me in the middle of the day. Someone had told him.

"Why didn't you tell me?" he wanted to know.

"Tell you what?"

"About the baby."

"Oh, *that* . . ."

"That! Laura, are you all right? I'll come right home. . ."

"No, no, wait!" and I heard myself saying, "There's no hurry, darling. It won't be for another seven months . . ."

I hung up. Seven months? Now, look what you've done, I scolded myself. Where are you going to get a baby by the end of seven months? Why not the whole nine? You need all the time you can get, Idiot! I counted on my fingers. May. A nice month to have a baby. Idiot! You'll have to throw yourself down a flight of stairs along about Christmas. Fall on the ice, maybe. Oh, this isn't really happening. Gladys Henning's shower never was. JP didn't just phone. Idiot!

I really did mean to confess as soon as JP came home that night. He brought flowers and he swung me around in a fit of emotion and we dined out to celebrate. He was so excited that I hadn't the heart to tell him the truth right then, so I waited until he went into the bathroom and when I heard the shower running full force, I called out in a moderately loud voice,

"JP, it's not true. We're not having a baby."

"That's wonderful, honey," he shouted from the shower.

Is it my fault he didn't hear me?

Well, it didn't stop there. We had to phone my mother and JP's mother and JP let the news filter through the office and, of course, all our friends and neighbors had to be told. The only one who wasn't aware of the little drama was the principal player in it, that wonderful man, Dr Broadbent. I decided to call on him once more. I didn't have much hope, but people did expect me to be seeing him, so I chose a day and a time for my appointment when I was sure someone I knew would be there, too. I even arranged to meet Gladys for lunch before our appointments. She remarked how lucky I was not to suffer from nausea as she had in her early months. I said it did bother me a little and, reluctantly, I waived the dessert.

Dr Broadbent was cordial. He remembered me but he was puzzled as to why I was there. I considered telling him the whole story, but I was sure he'd want to have me locked up, so I made up some symptoms. He smiled and nodded his head and, after having me weighed and my blood pressure checked, he patted me on the back and told me to come back in a month.

Wow! Had I fooled him, too?

After that, it became easier to pretend. I would have to put on some extra weight, so I indulged in gooey sundaes and rich desserts when I was alone, and in company with friends or when JP was home, I'd feign lack of appetite or nausea and pretend to be watching my weight. I let them pamper me and when JP wondered when I was going to get cravings for special foods, I sent him out one midnight for a pastrami sandwich. He didn't mind, though; he felt as though he was participating.

I bought some maternity clothes. I even enjoyed wearing them. I did put on weight but (and I suppose it was meant to be a compliment), everybody said I was carrying beautifully and that I didn't even *show*.

I managed one more appointment with Dr Broadbent, but on that occasion, he became impatient with me.

"Mrs Willis, how long are you going to go on with this?"

"Well," I said, counting on my fingers, "I figure I have four months left."

"And then what?"

"Then, I'll have my baby."

"Mrs Willis, you're not going to have a baby."

"Then, I'll have a miscarriage."

"What!"

"I've got to have this pregnancy," I told him. "I can't call it off now."

I saw his brow wrinkle and his eyes narrow suspiciously, but I got the drop on him. He wasn't slapping me into a straight jacket. Not yet, anyway. I gave in.

"I guess you're right."

He relaxed.

"Of course I'm right, dear lady. It isn't too late to say it was a mistake. Why don't you talk it over with your husband. He'll understand."

He put his arm around my shoulder and led me out of his office.

Okay, so he wouldn't help. For about half a minute, I considered going to JP and telling him the whole sad story, but in the other half of that minute, I saw his disappointment. I saw myself losing him. I said nothing and once a month I toddled to the doctor's office (actually to the movies). In my sixth month, I developed shortness of breath and in the seventh, heartburn, and in the eighth, false labor. And when the girls gave me a baby shower, I bubbled with joy and expressed delight with each bit of baby finery I unwrapped.

"When?" they asked.

"Soon," I promised.

Life had never been so happy. JP treated me like a queen. Our moments of love together were beautifully laced with a tenderness I'd never known from him before. When he held me in his arms, it was with a gentle care for me and our baby that bound us as a family. At least in his mind our baby existed and I could not destroy that. We found ourselves in love, romantic love, and we behaved like irresponsible adolescents, making love with a new excitement, an urgency that sent us to the bedroom whenever one of us smiled.

One night, as we lay entwined in each other's arms, JP said,

"One of these days we'll have to give up - this."

"This? You mean making love?"

"Uh-huh."

"Why? Are you sick of making love to a fat lady?"

"Never," he said, hugging me fondly. "I love my fat lady. I meant because of the baby. Maybe we shouldn't . . ."

"I'll ask Dr Broadbent," I promised, and the next day I told him that Dr B said making love would never hurt that baby. Which was certainly not a lie.

I was almost happy. If only it could have gone on like that, but it couldn't, of course. When JP wanted to buy a crib and stock up on Pampers, I had to think fast.

"It's bad luck," I said.

"What is?"

"Buying a crib."

"Who said?"

"You don't buy a crib, you borrow one."

"Aw, come on . . ."

"Betty offered," I said. "I couldn't hurt her feelings."

That kept JP from buying the crib but then I had to get to Betty and ask if she'd lend me the one she had in her attic. She said sure but she was surprised we didn't want to buy a brand new one, it being our first baby and all.

JP insisted on painting the small room even though I thought we should wait to see if it should be pink or blue. He said yellow would do for either sex and besides he wanted to have all the painting finished by the time the baby came. JP is a perfectionist and, of course, he wouldn't let me help.

When I saw him knocking himself out for a baby that was never going to be, I lost it. I locked myself in our bedroom and refused to talk to him. I decided the best thing to do was to go out by the window, leaving a note behind, and to disappear into some far-away place where he'd never hear of me again. For some unaccountable reason, I wanted to phone my sister, Amy, the one in Georgia, the one who'd been blessed with five kids of her own, the one who couldn't make it to my wedding, the one I hadn't seen in five years. When I lifted the receiver, I heard JP on the kitchen extension talking to someone.

"It's nothing, JP." I recognized Betty's voice. "Pregnant women do peculiar things sometimes. Just be gentle . . ."

"You're sure I shouldn't call the doctor?" JP said. I held my breath.

"No, of course not," Betty said. "Just sit tight. She'll be okay. Don't worry about it, JP."

Poor JP, I thought. How unfair this is to him. How did I ever get us into this mess? Well, I decided it was time to get us out of it. The consequences didn't matter. I would go out there and tell JP the whole truth. I flung open the door and cried,

"JP, let's move!"

"What?"

"Away from here. Out of town. Out west, maybe. When all this comes out, we'll never be able to hold our heads up . . ."

But JP was still under the influence of Betty's good advice, so he just put his arm around me and said everything was going to be all right and that I mustn't worry. It really wouldn't have made any difference what I told him at that point, he wouldn't have believed me anyway. All I could do was sit there and cry while JP, with his arm around me, tapped out a comforting there-there-there on my back.

In my ninth month, my mother phoned every other night. Her bag was packed and she was just waiting for the word and she'd come to look after JP while I was in the hospital and to care for us, me and the baby, when we came home. Pretty soon, I knew, I'd have to stage my *accident*. I wasn't quite sure how I would manage it, especially without Dr Broadbent's help. I'd have to try to make a deal with him to put me in the hospital for some alleged test or other and hang a "no visitors" sign on my door. I could offer him big money for his trouble. I'd already "paid" him a considerable sum in the pseudo checks I'd written to him. If he would agree, I could walk into the hospital, unhysterical, in the middle of the morning, alone. I couldn't have JP there, acting like an expectant father and the nurses thinking he was crazy. It meant one more visit to Dr Broadbent. He was astonished to see me.

"It's time," I told him.

"Mrs Willis, you can't be serious," he said. "You don't expect me to cooperate in this foolishness . . ."

I remained calm. I outlined my scheme - the hospital, tests, no visitors, etc., and I suggested that it would be well worth his while. He arose from his chair slowly, controlling quite well, I thought, an urge to strike me.

"Go home, Mrs Willis," he said. "I can't possibly do what you ask. Perhaps," he added, "perhaps counseling would help . . ."

What happened afterwards is a little vague. I went home and for the next few days, I moved about in a fog. I supposed I was really losing my mind. Then, yesterday, I think it was, I awoke early in the morning and I was terribly ill. I hauled myself out of bed and found, to my dismay, that my legs wouldn't support me and I slumped to the floor. When I came to, I saw JP in his pajamas with the phone in his hand, talking to someone who was giving him a hard time.

"But I tell you, Dr Broadbent, her labor has begun." He glanced at me and added, "She's writhing in pain on the floor!"

I writhed on cue. I heard him say okay and he hung up the phone and lifted me off the floor.

"It's all right, honey," he kept saying. "We'll make it in time. Be calm." And as he drew on his socks, he muttered, "Imagine that jerk of a doctor saying you weren't having a baby!"

It seemed like a dream, the climax of this nightmare I'd started so many months ago, but I was too ill to care. Somehow, JP got me into the car and we were off to the hospital. They put me into a wheelchair and hurried me away from poor JP who looked, as I glimpsed him from behind the closing elevator doors, as though everyone had run out on him.

Hours, or maybe only minutes later I was looking into the face of Dr Broadbent, a smiling, patient face, full of bedside manner. I fantasized that the dream would end with the announcement of a bouncing baby boy. Instead, I heard Dr Broadbent's voice delivering instructions and the only words I could make out were *no visitors*.

That was yesterday. I am confined to bed in this hospital room. I have refused to see anyone, not even JP or my mother. But I will have to see them sooner or later. And I think *now* I can. You see, Dr Broadbent has told me that I am pregnant - phenomenally, miraculously, delightfully and positively pregnant. It won't be easy, but I'm sure it won't be as difficult as the *first* nine months.

~ *Artichoke* ~
An Allegory

Not so very long ago, there nestled in a fine fertile valley, the fruitful kingdom of Artichoke, so called because its main industry was the growing, preserving and marketing of artichokes. It was a most productive kingdom and a very happy one, for all the people loved their work and each other.

Over this happy land reigned a paternal king and his devoted queen, the joy of whose lives was their daughter, soon to be sixteen, the lovely Princess Alahn.

Besides being Artichoke's gross national product, the fruit itself was a delicacy which the people relished at every meal. They never grew tired of it. So inured to its culture was the artichoke that it commanded a respect that other cultures reserved for religion. And, as it is with religions, there were certain strictures and ceremonials to be observed. In a land of such happiness and love, there was little need for rules, but there was one custom that everyone respected, one commandment that all obeyed. It applied to all the female children of the kingdom and it was: *Thou shalt not taste of the Artichoke until thou hast matured sixteen years.*

But wait . . . Although she was born restricted, a baby girl, from the day of her birth, was protected and revered as a special blessing. The more daughters that graced a family, the more esteemed were the parents. For every baby girl was born beautiful and she grew even more so with each passing day. Artichokians believed that the delicate beauty of the female child was a tenuous blessing, to be nurtured and only finally secured after sixteen years of sacrificial abstinence from the beloved artichoke. Consequently, the Artichokian Commandment was strictly adhered to. Woe betide the person who sought to tempt a young maid to the fruit prematurely. Few would dare, for the penalty was severe. History records but three cases in which each suspect died of suffocation following the amputation of his nose.

So, more important than even her wedding day, was a young girl's sixteenth birthday, her Artichoke Day, the highlights of which were two:

First, and most important, was the ceremonial reception of her first artichoke. It meant that she was fully matured, completely vested as an Artichokian, privileged thereafter, as her male counterpart was at birth, to imbibe, indulge and gratify herself with artichokes at will.

The second event was The Parade of Swains. Now, fully matured and capable of decision, the young woman could choose her husband from among all the eligible males in the land. How each one made her choice remained forever a mystery, respected and unquestioned, for in Artichoke, everyone loved everyone else and it made no difference who married whom. Still, the choice was the prerogative of the female, not the male, and the couple always lived happily ever after.

On the day of her maturing, her Artichoke Day,

the young girl would rise at dawn and dress, attended by her female friends and family members. Traditionally, her gown would be the pale yellow-green of the tenderest heart of artichoke. Her childhood braids would be loosed and her hair would be coiffed elegantly atop her head, signifying that she was leaving childhood behind. She was given gifts of jewelry and perfume, accoutrements denied her as a child. And when at last she appeared, radiant and smiling, the festival would begin.

There would be artichoke wine and artichoke soup, casseroles of artichoke *divan,* fresh, warm loaves of artichoke bread and artichoke *flan* for dessert. There would be games for the children, prizes and gifts; and for the adults, wining, dining and dancing throughout the day. The highlight of the festivities would come at the solemn moment when the young girl's parents would lead her to the seat of honor and with all eyes upon her, she would taste her first artichoke. Then and only then was she confirmed a woman. Finally, at day's end, the guests would return to their tables and The Parade of Swains would begin. The eligible young men would formally present themselves and she would choose from among them the one she would marry. Once she had selected her husband, there would be more celebration and plans would commence for her wedding.

Now, even more beautiful than all the others was Alahn, the daughter of the king and queen. With great excitement, the entire kingdom anticipated the celebration of her sixteenth birthday. Not only was she graceful, gifted and bright, but a princess, and the mate she chose would become, by marriage, a prince.

Naturally, each family with an eligible son was hopeful. From his birth, each boy had been groomed for the princess's Artichoke Day, toward the fulfillment of the family's dream that Alahn might lead him to the throne.

On the day of her festival, Alahn seemed to her glowing parents even more beautiful. She was splendidly gowned in cloth of artichoke gold, her shimmering hair piled high and braided with pearls. The princess, seeing her reflection in the mirror, was stunned by her own dazzlilng portrait - until she perceived that there was something wrong. There, clinging to the lid of one blue eye, was a tear. She dabbed at it with her new lace handkerchief, only to find that the tear would not be blotted away. Her parents, her friends, yea, all the kingdom were bewildered. Alas, Alahn could not tell them why the tear clung there.

"I am happy," she said. "I do not want to weep."

The king summoned the wizard who gazed into the princess's beautiful face with one lovely tear coursing through its smile, and he consoled her anxious parents.

"It is only with joy that she weeps, for she has beauty and health and wit and charm and blessings beyond the dreams of any maid."

And so, the king ordered the festival to begin.

The banquet hall was resplendent with crystal and flora. Princess Alahn reigned at the head of a grand table, her parents by her side. The king proudly raised a toast to his daughter and all the people cheered.

At last came the solemn moment when Alahn would be served her first artichoke. A hush fell upon the great hall as the steward set the golden dish before her, reverently lifting the cover to reveal the magnificent fruit. A murmur ran through the crowd as, with her regal fingers, she plucked the first delicate petal, dipped it into the golden butter and brought it to her lips. Then, as everyone watched, her lovely face contorted in a loathesome grimace, *she spit it out.*

Shocked, everyone began to talk at once.

"There is something wrong with the princess!"

"She has spit out the artichoke!"

The king and queen were dismayed and the princess, because she had offended everyone, gave way to a flood of tears.

Again, the wizard was summoned and after a brief consultation, the king announced that the princess was ill and must take to her bed. He invited them to continue their feasting but, alas, The Parade of Swains would have to be delayed until another time.

After a while, the princess recovered and was soon herself again. Except for one thing: she did not like, could not, would not eat artichoke. This was a very serious matter. The wizard was called again.

"Are you sure," he asked, "that Alahn is really sixteen? Perhaps you have made a mistake in the year of her birth and she is not yet matured."

The queen shook her head. There was no doubt about the princess's birth date; she was, indeed sixteen. The princess herself was contrite, but adamant.

"Dear parents," she said, "my heart is sad to so distress you, but I cannot control my taste. You have seen how a taste of artichoke distorts my face. Can you imagine how bitterly it violates my stomach?"

"Perhaps, in time," they hoped, for in every other respect, their daughter was normal, yea, perfect.

At last, The Parade of Swains was announced and all the young men came forth, dressed in their best and prepared to demonstrate their talents. Musicians brought their lyres and lutes; merchants their finest gifts; soldiers came and sailing men; came students of law and medicine; came artists, teachers and farmers' sons. Each one, privately, would have his moment to try to capture the princess's heart.

In the throne room, the king and queen waited anxiously, measuring each man's chances by the length of time the princess granted him. The Parade, which had been expected to last over a period of days, came to an end quickly as each swain was turned away. At last, the princess, understandably weary, emerged from her chamber and announced that the screening was over.

"Alas, dear parents," she said, smiling through her tear. "Each of the swains is more ugly than the other. Have you never noticed it before, that each man's nose resembles an artichoke?"

Astonished, the queen beheld her husband and saw for the first time that his nose did indeed resemble an artichoke. Bewildered, she beseeched her daughter,

"My darling, it is the nature of men to have such noses."

"But," protested the princess, "I find them repulsive. I do not choose to spend my life gazing into a face with an artichoke nose."

"But you must marry," insisted her father, the king. "Every woman must have a husband to care for her."

"But why?" Alahn asked. "I can care for myself."

"It is unnatural," pronounced the wizard.

"Then, I am an unnatural woman," said the

princess, and turning to her parents, she asked, "Can you love me still?"

Tearfully, the king and queen embraced their daughter, reassuring her of their love. And when they looked again into her face, the tear was gone.

"You see," she said, "I have much to be joyful of - parents who love me and a face that is not flawed by an artichoke nose."

When the people heard the shocking news of the princess's chauvinistic behavior, they formed a protest march to banish her from the kingdom. And though it broke the hearts of the king and queen, Alahn folded up her velvets and lace and stored them away in the royal closet, never to use them again. Wearing blue jeans and a leather jacket, she left Artichoke forever.

EPILOGUE

The scandal rocked through the kingdom with devastating results for, although the adult population was satisfied that the princess was gone, the young girls in the kingdom looked into their mirrors and their minds and discovered their independence. They began to steal into the larder and taste the artichokes, defying the stricture, eschewing the maturity ritual and deciding for themselves whether they liked or disliked artichokes. And those who liked them, stayed; but many more followed the princess into exile and, in time, as you might expect, the population of Artichoke dwindled to extinction.

~ Birthday Party ~
4 February 96

A Life in One Act

~Dramatis Personæ ~

Dear. . . . . . Husband
Fjus . . . . . . Mother
Father . . . . . . .Father
Poose . . . . . . .Brother
Sue . . . . . . .Sister
Nan. . . . . . .Sister

Time: Eternity
Place: Heaven

❧

Dear	Look at her - she's having another birthday.
Sue	She has two a year, as I recall, I always sent a card on *May* 4.
Dear	How old is she? I never could keep track.
Fjus	I forget. She was always changing things - her name, her birthday, her age . . .
Poose	Well, she's two years older than I'd be - seventy-two - so that makes her seventy-four.

Dear	She looks pretty good for seventy-four.
Fjus	I always thought she looked like Liz Taylor.
Dear	I thought she was better-looking than Liz.
Nan	*She* thought so, too. She thought she was the star of the family.
Father	First-borns are like that. We expect them to shine, so they do. You were all stars to me.
Poose	We did our best to shine. In school, *she* got the best grades. But we also found excuses to do our worst. Now, the worst is forgiven and only the best shines on.
Sue	When she told me she was a *writer*, I said, *Isn't everyone?*
Fjus	We're still waiting for that great American novel she promised.
Dear	Oh, she wrote it all right. It was called *Maxima Culpa* - Most Grievous Fault. It wouldn't fly today. Came close, but didn't fly then, either.
Nan	She was so *right* about everything. Once I sent her a letter and she sent it back with all my mistakes corrected.
Dear	She always regretted that.
Father	She may have known how to spell, but she had a block about math. I worried about that. Good thing she could type.
Fjus	Once, she was an executive secretary. I thought that was the top. When she became a writer, I thought it was a demotion.

Dear	That writing job was a turning point. *She* started making the plays. She'd always looked to me for the answers. I was losing control, so I guess I became something of a tyrant.
Fjus	You were always good to me. We were friends.
Poose	You helped me through college. You were my best man. And, no matter what, you were *her* inspiration, *her* guide, *her* support.
Dear	*Du mein Gedanke, du mein Sein und Herzen. Ich liebe dich.* I didn't say it in English. But she knew.
Nan	She's the last of us now. Of course, she *would* be the survivor.
Dear	I wasn't easy to live with, especially in those last years. I had emphysema. I didn't know I also had Alzheimer's. When she moved us to a new house, I got lost. One good thing, though: she got religion - well, her own made-up version of it. Now, she has her own space - she can ply all her hobbies.
Nan	Did any of you know *I* also did crafts?
Sue	And *I*, too had some skills.
Poose	Remember me? I was a Marine. After the war, I became a sales exec. I sold the first computer - *Univac* - to *Reader's Digest.*
Father	My forte was accounting.
Fjus	I was the only one of ten in my family who finished high school.

Dear	I was a teacher. An idea man. I wrote and crafted learning tools long before electronics got the message. My grand opus was *The Power to Persuade*. And I sold it for peanuts.
Poose	Once, in rehab, they made me do a painting. I wonder what ever happened to it.
Dear	It doesn't matter. The world moves along without us. Only to *them* does it matter. They try to keep us with them with our things. I didn't leave much behind. She found my wad. *That* she didn't keep!
Fjus	She phoned me almost every day during my last few months. But she was in California on Mother's Day. She didn't call. I waited till she got home, though. She called and we had a long chat on the phone. I didn't want to hang up. She said she'd come to visit in a month or so. I knew she'd come sooner than that. The next day, I died.
Poose	She didn't handle our deaths very well. I was the first. At least we'd spent two good weeks together in Florida just before I left.
Nan	I was the last. Just a month ago. She didn't make it to my funeral. There was a big snowstorm in the east and she couldn't get to Ohio. Once, we had a bitter fight, said ugly things to each other. That was when

	Sue died. But it was more than grief - it was about a resentment I'd had all my life. We were sisters, but we were strangers. We patched it up before I left. I'm glad I didn't carry it to my grave.
Sue	So is she. I knew her a little better than you did. But she didn't intimidate me. *I* made some marks for myself. *I* had some trophies.
Nan	I had nine kids.
Dear	Look, she's trying to draw the baby, the new grandkid I didn't live to see. She used to practice her drawing on me.
Fjus	And on me. She did a snow scene for me. It hung over the server in the dinette.
Sue	Someone took it, probably for the frame.
Father	When she was a little girl, we thought she was talented. She drew, played the piano and wrote stories. I had to punish her for the stories, though; writing love stories at twelve wasn't appropriate.
Dear	We all made mistakes with our kids. She never thought her efforts measured up. Now, she's recovering, hurrying to do it all before her time is up.
Fjus	I always liked it when she sang in church. Now, she sings with a chorale.
Father	And she's joined the Art League.
Sue	Still doing crossword puzzles. And the Fan Club, whatever that is.

Nan	She has her kids.
Dear	And Doga, *my* dog.
Poose	Health, security, friends . . .
Dear	Her own way . . . She misses my presence in her life but not my control. I'm glad she wasn't there when the breathing stopped.
Fjus	We'll keep watching . . .
Father	. . . applaud when she scores. Be there when she misses.
Dear	So, go for it, Swid. Do it all!
Chorus	*Happy Birthday, Jude*

ॐ

ED. NOTE: This opus was transcribed from an actual dream.

MR AND SR